D1469294

Alkaline Diet for Beginners

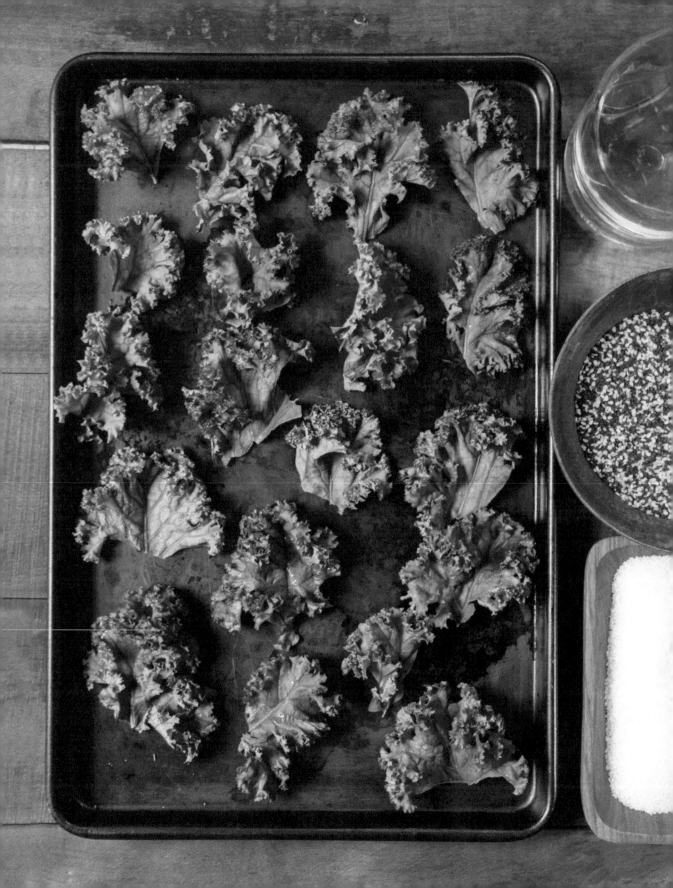

The Alkaline Diet
for Beginners

UNDERSTAND PH, EAT WELL, AND RECLAIM YOUR HEALTH

Jennifer Koslo, PhD, RDN, CSSD

ROCKRIDGE
PRESS

Copyright © 2016 by Rockridge Press, Berkeley, California

No part of this publication may be reproduced, stored in a retrieval system, or transmitted in any form or by any means, electronic, mechanical, photocopying, recording, scanning, or otherwise, except as permitted under Sections 107 or 108 of the 1976 US Copyright Act, without the prior written permission of the Publisher. Requests to the Publisher for permission should be addressed to the Permissions Department, Rockridge Press, 918 Parker St, Suite A-12, Berkeley, CA 94710.

Limit of Liability/Disclaimer of Warranty: The Publisher and the author make no representations or warranties with respect to the accuracy or completeness of the contents of this work and specifically disclaim all warranties, including without limitation warranties of fitness for a particular purpose. No warranty may be created or extended by sales or promotional materials. The advice and strategies contained herein may not be suitable for every situation. This work is sold with the understanding that the publisher is not engaged in rendering medical, legal, or other professional advice or services. If professional assistance is required, the services of a competent professional should be sought. Neither the Publisher nor the author shall be liable for damages arising herefrom. The fact that an individual, organization, or website is referred to in this work as a citation and/or potential source of further information does not mean that the author or the Publisher endorses the information the individual, organization, or website may provide or recommendations they/it may make. Further, readers should be aware that websites listed in this work may have changed or disappeared between when this work was written and when it is read.

For general information on our other products and services or to obtain technical support, please contact our Customer Care Department within the United States at (866) 744-2665, or outside the United States at (510) 253-0500.

Rockridge Press publishes its books in a variety of electronic and print formats. Some content that appears in print may not be available in electronic books, and vice versa.

TRADEMARKS: Rockridge Press and the Rockridge Press logo are trademarks or registered trademarks of Callisto Media Inc. and/or its affiliates, in the United States and other countries, and may not be used without written permission. All other trademarks are the property of their respective owners. Rockridge Press is not associated with any product or vendor mentioned in this book.

Cover photography © Stocksy/Martí Sans

Interior photography © Stockfood/Glasshouse Images, p.2; Stockfood/Gräfe & Unzer Verlag/Wolfgang Schardt, p.8; Shutterstock, p.14; Stocksy/Darren Muir, p.25; Stocksy/Martí Sans, p. 28; Stocksy/Ali Harper, p.31; Stockfood/Magdalena Hendey, p.40; Stockfood/Gräfe & Unzer Verlag/Fotos mit Geschmack, p.48; Stockfood/Charlie Richards, p.66; Stockfood/PhotoCuisine, p.78; Stockfood/ Gräfe & Unzer Verlag/mona binner PHOTOGRAPHIE, p.96; Stockfood/Great Stock!, p.114; Stockfood/Meike Bergmann, p.130; Stockfood/Gräfe & Unzer Verlag/mona binner, p.142.

ISBN: Print 978-1-62315-814-9
eBook 978-1-62315-815-6

Contents

Is the Alkaline Diet for You?

Have you ever wondered what the Alkaline Diet is and how it works, but have struggled to find straightforward answers? Proponents of the diet suggest that replacing acid-forming foods with alkaline foods in your diet can improve health, help you lose weight, and fight serious diseases like cancer. But is there any strong evidence behind the diet, and if so, who can benefit from following it?

Without getting too technical, our bodies maintain a delicate pH balance, and for good health, our bodies need to be slightly alkaline. Chapter 1 will cover everything you need to know about pH, but for now, know that the pH scale runs from 0 to 14—a pH over 7 is alkaline, and a pH lower than 7 is acidic. Now think of the Standard American Diet. Most people are bathing their cells in an acid bath by making poor choices several times a day by eating processed carbs, refined sugar, alcohol, factory-farmed red meat, fried and fatty foods, and full-fat dairy products. This type of diet takes a toll on the body, especially the digestive system, liver, and kidneys, and can result in chronic health problems such as hypertension, cancer, and renal disease.

Conversely, by filling your plate with alkaline-forming foods like leafy greens, veggies, fruits, sprouted grains, almonds, beans, root vegetables, and some tubers, you feed your body and cells vitamins, minerals, fiber, water, antioxidants, and phytochemicals that can provide protection from disease. Simply put, healthy food creates healthy cells and junk creates junk. As a general rule of thumb, if you want to follow an alkaline diet, 80 percent of what you eat should be alkalizing foods and the remaining 20 percent acid-forming foods. A superb array of high-alkaline recipes, starting on page 42, will make sure you're never bored and always satisfied with your meals.

If at first this all sounds overwhelming, take heart. Following a more alkaline diet means choosing fruits, vegetables, plant proteins, healthy fats, and whole, unprocessed foods over prepared and highly processed foods that generally contain far too much sodium, unhealthy fats, and other additives. You won't have to count calories or cut out whole food groups; you just need to become familiar with which foods are more alkaline forming and which are more acid forming. If given a list of foods, most people could put them in the acid or alkaline group the majority of the time: Eat the foods you *know* are good for you, and stay away from the foods you *know* are bad for you.

So who can benefit, and is there any evidence to support this type of eating plan? The Alkaline Diet is for anyone who wants to decrease their risk for chronic diseases like hypertension, stroke, and type 2 diabetes; minimize their risk for kidney stones; or simply move toward a more plant-based eating style. While not designed for weight loss, this can be an added bonus for most people following the Alkaline Diet. Eating whole, unprocessed foods means eating lots of fiber-packed veggies, fruits, and beans, which boost satiety (that satisfied feeling signaling you've had enough), so you shouldn't be hungry on this diet. In chapter 1, you will find out how a few simple food substitutions and additions can correct your acid-base woes and steer your diet in the direction of good health.

Of course, to get the full benefits of the Alkaline Diet, it is also important to include a program of regular exercise, get a sufficient amount of quality sleep, hydrate, and include daily stress-reducing activities in your schedule.

Look at your plate and peek in your glass. What direction are you moving on the pH scale?

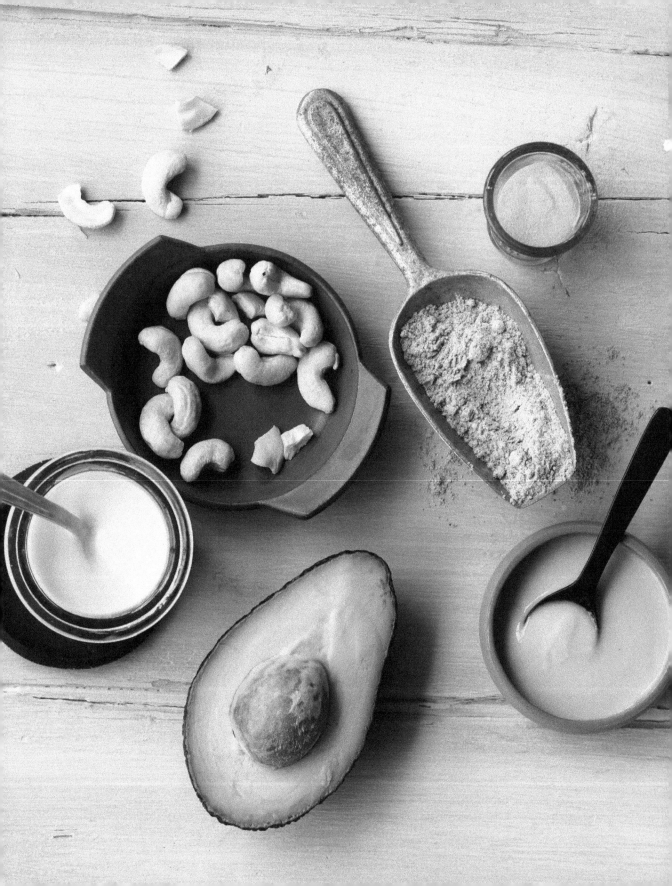

CHAPTER ONE

Let's Talk Basics

The Alkaline Diet is based on the acid/alkaline theory of disease. When we break down the foods we eat and extract the energy (calories) from them, we are actually burning the foods, but in a slow and controlled fashion. Just like burning wood in a furnace, when you burn foods, they produce waste products, sometimes called "ash." This ash can be acidic or alkaline, depending on the protein, sulfur, or mineral content of the food. Eating foods that leave behind a lot of acidic ash, such as refined carbs, sugar, and fried or processed foods, can over time increase inflammation in the body, leaving us vulnerable to disease.

The body includes a number of organ systems that are adept at neutralizing and eliminating acid, but there is a limit to how much acid even a healthy body can cope with effectively. The premise of the Alkaline Diet is not to change your blood pH, but rather to remove the stress of maintaining a healthy pH by giving your body the tools it needs to thrive. Alkaline-forming foods, including whole fruits, vegetables, tubers, and plant proteins, are alkaline because they are fresh, natural, anti-inflammatory, delicious foods rich in vitamins, minerals, chlorophyll, and antioxidants.

What Is pH?

Let's start with a mini-chemistry refresher on pH and what it means. Simply put, pH is a measurement of the hydrogen ion concentration in the body. The term *pH* stands for "power of hydrogen," where *p* is short for "potenz" (the German word for *power*) and *H* is the element symbol for hydrogen. The total pH scale ranges from 1 to 14, with 7 considered neutral. A pH less than 7 is acidic, and solutions with a pH greater than 7 are basic or alkaline.

For good health, our bodies need to be slightly alkaline, and the pH of our blood and other important cellular fluids is designed to be at a pH of 7.365 to 7.45. But it's important to note that the pH value varies greatly within the body. Some parts are acidic, and others are alkaline; there is no set level. The stomach is loaded with hydrochloric acid, giving it a pH value between 2 and 3.5 (highly acidic), which is necessary to break down the foods we eat and to kill harmful bacteria. Saliva ranges from a pH of 6.8 to 7.4, and your skin is acidic (pH 4 to 6.5) to act as a protective barrier to the environment. Urine has a variable pH from acid to alkaline, depending on your body's need to balance your internal environment as a result of the foods you eat.

By far, the most important measurement is your blood pH. Keeping it in that narrow range of 7.365 to 7.45 may seem simple enough, but rather than operating on a mathematical scale, pH operates on a logarithmic scale with multiples of 10.

Therefore, it takes 10 times the amount of alkalinity to neutralize an acid. For example, a jump from 6 to 7 doesn't seem like a lot, but in reality, it will take 10 times the amount of alkalinity to neutralize that range. A pH of 5 is 100 times more acidic than pH 7, and pH 4 is 1,000 times more acidic. Get the idea?

Now, before you start stressing about falling out of range, take heart in knowing that your body is generally awesome at tightly regulating the pH of your blood. But it doesn't just "find" the balance; it has a number of mechanisms to do this and will maintain the pH of your blood between 7.365 and 7.45 *no matter what.* When you make poor diet and lifestyle choices, your body has to work harder to maintain this balance. Addressing acidity and inflammation in your body by shifting the majority of your dietary choices to alkaline-forming foods is fundamental to balancing your system and bringing your body back to vitality.

How Food Affects Your Body

Researchers have known for years that the composition of the diet can strongly affect the acid-base balance of the body. Diet-induced changes in the acidity of the urine have long piqued the interest of physiologists because they demonstrate the kidneys' role in the maintenance of homeostasis, or a state of balance in the body. Paleolithic researchers point out the drastic changes in our diets compared to that of our hunter-gatherer ancestors and the concomitant rise in chronic diseases.

Author and journalist Michael Pollan's guideline that people should "eat food, not too much, mostly plants," is often quoted, but less often followed. According to a new study published in the *British Medical Journal,* more than half of Americans' calories come from "ultra-processed foods" devoid of valuable nutrients and shockingly high in sodium, added sugars, and unhealthy fats. The processed foods are then coupled with a high intake of acid-forming animal proteins and a low intake of fruits and vegetables. It's no surprise that this type of diet is a recipe for disease, but why? One reason is that the modern industrialized diet has exchanged potassium- and magnesium-rich foods (present in abundance in plant foods) for sodium chloride (salt). This displacement creates—among other things—a deficiency of potassium in the diet, increasing the net acid load in the body.

To make matters worse, over time, a high acid load produces what is called "low-grade chronic metabolic acidosis," which means we are chronically in a state of high acidity and inflammation. Because the body must at all costs operate at a stable pH, neutralizing a consistently high dietary acid load puts a strain on our bodies' natural buffering systems. The consequences of your body's attempt to maintain a constant pH in the face of an acidic environment are high concentrations of metabolic wastes, which can lead to muscle wasting and an increased risk for chronic disease.

Acute inflammation, such as your body responding to a fever or cut, is good and necessary for health. But chronic inflammation, a normal bodily process gone awry, has a domino effect that can seriously undermine your health. The good news is that what you put in your mouth affects your inflammation levels, and using foods, herbs, and spices to help reduce inflammation in the body is actually one of the best ways to protect your health.

According to the *European Journal of Nutrition,* scientific studies have now provided evidence showing that when acid-producing foods are minimized in the diet and replaced with alkaline-producing foods, this shift lowers acid levels and reduces the strain on your body's natural buffering systems. Reducing your acid load may then help prevent or delay the formation of kidney stones, maintain muscle mass, lower your risk for type 2 diabetes, and improve heart health by promoting a healthy blood pressure. Employing a few simple strategies to neutralize your high-acid diet may mean the difference between chronic low-grade acidosis and a healthy, disease-free body.

Health Conditions Improved By Eating a More Alkaline Diet

A study in the *British Journal of Nutrition* concludes that "the available research makes a compelling case that diet-induced acidosis is a real phenomenon, has significant clinical relevance, may largely be prevented through dietary changes, and should be recognized and treated." Here are a few conditions the Alkaline Diet can help prevent.

Hypertension, stroke, and heart disease
According to the Centers for Disease Control and Prevention, over 33 percent of adults have high blood pressure, a condition that increases the risk for heart disease and stroke. While there are a number of risk factors for high blood pressure and heart disease, including inactivity and being overweight, there is a clear and distinct link between what you eat and your risk. According to research published in *Clinical Nutrition*, the Standard American Diet, deficient in fruits and vegetables and containing excessive animal products, induces metabolic acidosis and a low urine pH. This high dietary acid load is more likely to result in hypertension and may increase the risk for hypertension and heart disease. ***Bottom Line:*** The Alkaline Diet is high in the minerals potassium and magnesium, which promote a healthy blood pressure. Eating more alkalizing foods can positively shift your mineral ratio and may decrease your risk for heart disease.

Kidney stones According to the National Kidney Foundation, 1 in 10 people will develop kidney stones over the course of a lifetime. While there are a number of risk factors, a diet high in animal protein, sodium, and sugar may significantly increase your risk by adding more "stone promoting" nutrients than your kidneys can filter. This is especially true with a high-sodium diet, which increases the amount of calcium your kidneys must filter. Stone promoters, including calcium, oxalate (certain nuts, chocolate), sodium, phosphorus, and uric acid (animal proteins), contribute to low-grade metabolic acidosis in the body. And while a young, healthy person can usually filter these stone promoters, as we age, we experience a normal decline in kidney function. Passing a kidney stone is no picnic, and now recent research published in the journal *Urological Research* has shown that dietary acid load is the best predictor of stone formation. ***Bottom Line:*** Adding more alkalizing, nutrient-rich foods to your diet can reduce the accumulation of stone promoters.

Muscle mass As we age, we naturally lose muscle mass, and more so if we lead an inactive lifestyle. Less muscle mass means we burn fewer calories during the day, contributing to the "weight creep" that most people experience as they age. More importantly, losing muscle mass makes us more susceptible to falls and fractures and a loss of independence. A study published in the *American Journal of Clinical Nutrition* found that an alkaline-rich diet high in fruits and vegetables reduced net acid load in elderly adults, resulting in preservation of muscle mass. ***Bottom Line:*** We all want to keep our independence as we age, and adding a serving of fruits and vegetables to each of your meals can help.

Type 2 diabetes The Centers for Disease Control and Prevention estimates that about 10 percent of the adult US population has type 2 diabetes, a metabolic disorder that causes your blood sugar to rise higher than normal and where your cells become resistant to the action of the hormone insulin to bring it back into balance. Type 2 diabetes is largely preventable, and recent research has found that dietary acid load is associated with increased risk. In a study published in *Diabetologia* in 2013, researchers conducted a 14-year cohort study analyzing dietary information collected from a questionnaire from almost 70,000 French women. From the responses, the researchers calculated the potential renal acid load (PRAL) and found a trend correlating a high dietary acid load to an increased risk for type 2 diabetes. *Bottom Line:* In conjunction with maintaining a healthy weight, scientific evidence shows that a dietary pattern that emphasizes alkaline foods may reduce the risk of type 2 diabetes.

Cancer and chemotherapy Although diet-induced acidosis may indeed increase cancer risk, at this time there is no clinical research that an alkaline diet can prevent cancer. However, according to the journal *Cancer*, preliminary studies have shown that by eating more alkaline-promoting foods, urine pH can be manipulated to optimize the effectiveness of chemotherapy drugs. If you have cancer or are undergoing chemotherapy, speak to your doctor and dietitian before making changes to your diet. *Bottom Line:* The American Cancer Society recommends consuming a healthy diet with an emphasis on plant foods, five to nine servings of fruits and vegetables each day, and a cap on consumption of sodium, alcohol, processed meat, and red meat, which is similar to the Alkaline Diet.

Chronic low back pain While research is still in its infancy, there is some evidence indicating that chronic low back pain improves with supplementation of alkaline minerals. A study published in the *Journal of Trace Elements in Medicine and Biology* showed that increasing magnesium through supplementation allowed for the proper function of enzyme systems and activation of vitamin D, which in turn improved back pain. *Bottom Line:* If you suffer from back pain, following the Alkaline Diet will boost your levels of magnesium and may ease your symptoms.

The Standard American Diet leaves much to be desired, leaving the body shortchanged on many essential vitamins and minerals. Left unchecked, in the short term, these shortages can make you feel tired, disrupt your sleep, wreak havoc on your mood and concentration, and lead to weight gain. In the long term, diet imbalances can lead to chronic diseases like high blood pressure, type 2 diabetes, heart disease, and kidney stones. Feeding your body with a mix of nutrient-dense foods on a daily basis gives it a fighting chance against disease.

ALKALINE WATER?

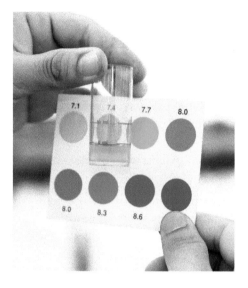

While researching the Alkaline Diet, you may have heard that alkaline water, water that is less acidic than tap water, is even better. Alkaline water is rich in alkalizing compounds including calcium, silica, potassium, magnesium, and bicarbonate. Normal tap water is generally neutral, with a pH of 7, and alkaline water has a pH of 8 or 9. Alkaline water can be bought in many grocery stores, and water ionizers are sold in many large chain stores as well. According to the Mayo Clinic, regular water is best for most people, as there is no scientific evidence that fully verifies the claims made by alkaline water proponents. Thus far, the current clinical research for claims that alkaline water helps treat chronic acidosis, improves overall health, protects us from toxins, improves gut health, and reduces liver damage is unconvincing. It is possible that drinking alkaline water may provide benefit to some people in some circumstances; however, studies have not produced hard evidence that doing so will benefit your health. People with kidney disease or who are taking certain medications that alter kidney function are cautioned against using it because the minerals in alkaline water could accumulate in their bodies. If you don't suffer from kidney problems, you may consider drinking some alkaline water. So far, water with naturally occurring minerals seems to be your best bet as an alkaline water source.

Alkaline Diet Frequently Asked Questions

There is a lot of conflicting information on the Alkaline Diet, so the following section is meant to answer some common questions as you get started on eating a more alkaline diet.

Is the Alkaline Diet gluten free? While the Alkaline Diet is not designed to specifically be gluten free, following it means excluding white flour–based products (wheat), barley, and most processed foods. You can still enjoy a number of nutrient-rich, alkalizing whole grains and seeds including amaranth, buckwheat, brown rice, millet, and quinoa, which are all gluten free.

Will I need to buy special, hard-to-find ingredients? That depends. Does your pantry include a bin of sweet potatoes and jars of dried beans? Is your refrigerator stocked with fresh fruits and vegetables? Do you keep an arsenal of fresh herbs and dried spices on hand? While these items are not hard to find, if you are just embarking on a more whole foods–based diet, then you may need to set aside some time to do a pantry overhaul.

Can I eat meat? If not, what are some protein-rich alkaline foods? The good news is that if you are a meat eater, you don't have to completely give it up to follow the Alkaline Diet. A key tenet of the Alkaline Diet is the 80/20 Rule (explained in depth on page 19), which means meat should not be the star of the show. And eat it sparingly, maybe two or three times a week instead of seven, emphasizing quality (hormone free) over quantity. Plant sources of protein are abundant on the Alkaline Diet, and you'll be meeting your needs by eating beans, lentils, nuts, and seeds. The recipes included in this book are free of animal ingredients.

Will I lose weight? The Alkaline Diet is not a low-calorie diet and is not designed specifically for weight loss. However, the body is designed to be alkaline, and one of the by-products of chronic metabolic acidosis is weight gain. Your body tends to readily store the same foods that are acidic including unhealthy fats and refined sugar. Conversely, alkaline-forming plants are high in filling fiber, adding volume and satiety to your meals so you end up eating less overall, which can bring your weight back to a healthy range.

How long will it take to get "alkaline?" This is a great question but one that is tough to answer. Everyone's body is different, and each person's diet prior to going alkaline is different. Plus, to keep things in perspective, the goal is not to strive to get a perfect pH reading on a daily basis. Rather, the goal of going alkaline is to increase your energy and move your body to a healthier state. If your diet has been pretty acidic, you may feel an impact within a day or two. If you are already eating fairly clean, your results may be more subtle, such as improved sleep or concentration.

Can I still eat out? Absolutely! You just have to do your research beforehand. The consumer demand for fresh, locally grown foods has resulted in the growth of restaurants that cater to a number of diets including vegan, vegetarian, and gluten free. The same foods on the Alkaline Diet can be found on the menus of establishments catering to health-conscious consumers.

Can my family and kids eat an Alkaline Diet with me? Again, the answer to this is a resounding YES! The Alkaline Diet is a balanced, health-promoting diet, adequate in calories and all essential nutrients to meet the nutritional needs of everyone— from young children to young adults to the elderly. There will be no need to cook separate meals when following the Alkaline Diet, and your whole family will reap the health benefits.

What about holidays? Holidays can be tricky for anyone eating clean, and so it is best to be proactive: Use the recipes in this book to take dishes to your gatherings to share with your friends and family. Create new traditions by swapping out your usual recipes for those that are alkaline producing, and you may find that this year's holiday eating doesn't add pounds to your waistline.

Is food preparation complicated and time-consuming? Think of your cooking and following an Alkaline Diet not as a chore but as an act of love for your family and your body. Take a fun approach that avoids a sense of drudgery from the start. Chapter 2 will give you all of the tips and tools you'll need to be most efficient with preparing your meals, including a 30-Day Meal Plan.

Do the foods on this diet taste good? The Alkaline Diet emphasizes fresh, whole, unprocessed foods bursting with flavor. By starting with a clean slate, you can retrain your taste buds and change your palate to love nutritious foods. Chapter 2 will provide tips for handling those particularly pesky cravings for unhealthy fats, salt, and sugar as you remove them from your diet.

Alkaline- and Acid-Forming Foods

While many foods obviously fall into an acid or alkaline category, others aren't quite as evident at first glance. Take a lemon, for example. You know a lemon tastes tart, so it must clearly be acidic, right? While the nature of a lemon is acidic, once it is metabolized by the body, it has an alkalizing effect. Foods that are acidic in nature are not always acid forming once they are consumed. Many acidic foods like citrus, kefir, and sauerkraut are healing and alkalizing. To add to the confusion, numerous charts on acidifying and alkalizing foods simply use the words "acid foods" and "alkaline foods," which really doesn't give an accurate picture.

According to the journal *Seminars in Dialysis,* to more accurately predict the acid or base potential of a given food, scientists worked long and hard and came up with a technique that takes into account the nutrient composition of the food and, in layman's terms, can determine what the true acid or base load on the body is. Thus was born the potential renal acid load (PRAL) scale. A negative PRAL score indicates the food is basic/alkaline. A positive PRAL score indicates the food is acidic. A score of 0 indicates the food is neutral. If you add the PRAL values for all the foods you eat in a day, you get the net acid or alkaline load. While it isn't necessary to micromanage your diet to get the lowest PRAL values, it may be interesting to calculate the PRAL values of your normal diet.

What Can and Cannot Be Affected By What You Eat

By now you might be intrigued about giving this Alkaline Diet a shot, but how can you really tell if it's working? The good news is that testing your pH is easy and cheap, and you can easily test your saliva and urine pH levels at home. Just head to the local drugstore and pick up a pack of pH test strips. In case you are met with a puzzled look from the clerk, it may help to ask for litmus paper; they are the same thing. You can also order them online from retailers like Amazon.

Understanding the Difference between Blood pH, Saliva pH, and Urine pH

Remember, you are not trying to change the pH of your blood. The pH reading you get when you test your urine or saliva is *not* the pH of your internal environment; it is the pH of the fluids that your body is eliminating. Your body needs to maintain your internal pH within a very narrow range of 7.365 to 7.45. The range you will find in your urine and saliva may vary widely as your body eliminates excess acids, which is necessary in order to maintain your internal pH within this narrow range.

The pH of the urine reveals how the body is working to maintain the proper pH of the blood. Urine testing indicates the efforts of the body via the kidneys, adrenals, and lungs to regulate pH through excreting acids and assimilating minerals, such as calcium, magnesium, sodium, and potassium. These minerals function as buffers to help maintain and balance your blood pH in that tight range. The ideal range for urine pH is between 6.5 and 7.5. If it is below 6.5, it may indicate your body's buffering system is overwhelmed.

While saliva uses buffers just like urine, it relies on this to a lesser degree and is more likely to contain acidic bacteria throughout the day. Testing your saliva may be more convenient than testing your urine, but keep in mind that urine is a better reflection of the processes the body is undertaking to remove acid from the body. An ideal range for saliva pH is between 7.0 and 7.5.

Because there are going to be fluctuations in the readings you get, it is recommended that you take the average of several readings of urine and/or saliva pH to gain a bigger picture of your progress rather than concentrating on each reading in isolation. You are looking for *trends* that you can follow so that you can notice the difference any changes in your diet make.

And remember that the pH scale is logarithmic, meaning that each step is 10 times the previous. For example, a pH of 4.5 is 10 times more acidic than a pH of 5.5, which is 100 times more acidic than a pH of 6.5. And to give you some perspective, a person eating a Standard American Diet may have saliva and urine pH readings of less than 6.0.

Testing Urine and Saliva pH

Testing your pH takes less than a minute, and it is a great way to gather baseline data, track your progress in boosting your alkalinity, and keep motivated to stay on track. But it has to be done correctly.

HOW TO TEST

Testing your saliva pH Testing your saliva as soon as you wake up and before you do anything else will give you the most accurate result. If this isn't convenient, wait at least two hours after eating or brushing your teeth to take your measurement. To do this, fill your mouth with saliva and then swallow it. Repeat this step again to ensure your spit is clean, and then place some saliva on the pH strip. Write down the pH number along with the date and time to monitor your progress.

Testing your urine pH Just like saliva, your first urination of the day will give you the most accurate picture and measure of your body's overnight metabolic work. You can test your urine pH by either urinating directly on the pH strip or by collecting urine in a cup and dipping the paper into the urine. Write down the pH number, date, and time to monitor your progress.

INTERPRETING THE VALUES

As the test paper is moistened, it will take on color. The color relates to the acid or alkaline state of your saliva or urine and ranges from yellow to dark blue. Match the color of your test strip with the chart provided on the back of your test kit.

Your saliva pH will tell you how effective your body is at dealing with the acidic foods you may have eaten the day and night before and how well the salivary glands are performing in dealing with excess acidity in the diet. Your urine pH will be an indication of how your body's alkaline buffering system is working to neutralize the acids you have consumed as well as those that have been produced overnight through metabolism.

Goal pH The ideal urine reading should be between 6.5 and 7.5, and saliva readings should be between 7.0 and 7.5.

WHAT A CHANGE INDICATES

Remember that at first, most people will have readings below 6.5 due to the acid-forming tendency of the Standard American Diet. That's okay! Simply work toward filling your glass with fresh water and your plate with more vegetables, fruits, root vegetables, nuts, seeds, and spices. Strive to get 80 percent of your nutrition from these nutrient-dense alkalizing foods, a goal known as the 80/20 Rule.

The 80/20 Rule

Getting healthy is not about trying to be perfect out of the gates or depriving yourself of the foods you really love. Success in "going alkaline" and sustaining this lifestyle (note the use of the word *lifestyle* as opposed to *diet*) is about moderation, because life is all about balance. Deprivation is the cause for most diet failures, and finding a perfect balance can be challenging and confusing at first. To reap the most benefits of the Alkaline Diet, employ the 80/20 Rule. What this means is that to maintain a healthy internal environment, you should aim to eat a diet that consists of about 80 percent alkaline-forming foods, with the remaining 20 percent being acid-forming foods. In general, animal proteins and refined starches are acid, and most beans, vegetables, and fruits are alkaline.

It's easy to put this into practice if you think in terms of food groups and visualize your plate: For optimal health, fruits, vegetables, tubers, healthy fats, and plant proteins should take up 80 percent of your plate, and starches and other acidic foods should make up the last 20 percent. If you do this at each meal and snack, this guarantees your diet will be 80 percent alkaline and 20 percent acid. You may be tempted to eliminate acid-forming foods entirely from your diet. However, this would be a mistake. Even though high-protein foods such as meat, milk, fish, and some beans are acidifying, your body needs protein to rebuild and repair.

So if you love tofu (PRAL -0.3), which is a low-acid/mildly alkaline food, then go ahead and include it in your diet in moderation. And while it's not a high-protein food, you can even include a piece of chocolate or birthday cake once in a while. The key is balance and moderation and shifting your diet from an overreliance on acid-forming foods to one where they start to take up a smaller and smaller part of your plate. Slowly add the foods that will have the most powerful impact, and before you know it, the good will outweigh the bad and your health and energy will go to the next level.

Acid-Forming Foods to Avoid

When it comes to restoring the pH balance in your body, it's beneficial to know which foods to embrace and which ones to avoid. A food's acid-forming tendency in the body has nothing to do with the actual pH of the food itself. Rather, foods are classified depending on the minerals they release into the urine. As you are starting out, use the following list to make personal decisions about which acid-forming foods to include in your 20 percent or exclude entirely.

Alcohol Even a small amount of alcohol has an effect on your body. When you drink, alcohol is absorbed directly into your bloodstream and distributed throughout your body, where it remains until the liver processes it. Of the four macronutrients, three—protein, carbohydrates, and fat—can be stored in our bodies, but the fourth, alcohol, cannot. For this reason, it takes priority over everything else in order to be metabolized: doing so means that all of the other processes that should be taking place are interrupted. Devoid of nutrients, alcohol is viewed as a toxic waste by your body and should be used in moderation.

Caffeine Have you ever thought about what is actually going on in your body when you throw back that energy drink or sip that coffee? Caffeine, like alcohol, quickly enters your bloodstream, and it only takes 45 minutes for 99 percent of it to be absorbed through the membranes of your mouth, throat, and stomach. Chemically speaking, caffeine is basic, but coffee, tea, caffeinated energy drinks, hot chocolate, and cola are classified as acid-forming due to other chemicals present, such as phosphorus and formic and acetic acids. After absorption, the liver metabolizes caffeine and the by-products

are filtered by the kidneys and exit the body with urine. To reduce the work of your liver, aim to switch your regular cup of coffee for some nourishing herbal tea or a tall glass of sparkling water.

Animal products Animal proteins, including meat, eggs, and dairy, are considered some of the most highly acid-forming foods you can eat. And in the United States, people in general eat far too much animal protein, centering meals around it rather than using it as a side. Animal proteins are typically high in unhealthy saturated fats and cholesterol, and unless they are organic, they may contain hormones and antibiotics. Meat and eggs contain a lot of sulfur-containing amino acids that are metabolized into sulfuric acid, which must be buffered by the body with calcium compounds, putting additional strain on your kidneys. Your body needs sufficient protein for repair and recovery, so you don't want to eliminate protein sources entirely; you just want to balance out your choices and emphasize those that are alkaline-forming more often. On the alkaline diet, you will get plenty of fiber-packed, nutrient-rich plant protein by swapping out your meat several times a week for beans and legumes.

Refined sugars Americans eat *far* too much sugar and, like sodium, it is ubiquitous in our food supply. The average American eats about 22 teaspoons of sugar a day, which adds up to more than 70 pounds a year.

Compare this to the current recommendations to limit added sugars to 5 teaspoons per day for adult women and 8 to 9 teaspoons per day for adult men. Eating too much sugar can lead to unhealthy weight gain, high blood sugar, diabetes, and high cholesterol. The major sources of added sugars are acid-forming foods including soft drinks, candy, cakes, cookies, and dairy desserts. Use the Nutrition Facts panel on your food labels to add up the sugar you consume in a day to get a baseline of your intake. Fresh foods do not contain added sugars, so stick to eating the natural nutrient-rich sugars that nature intended us to eat.

Grains The top grains consumed in the United States, corn and wheat, are considered highly acidic. After they are consumed and metabolized in the body, they produce acids that must be eliminated by the liver. Wheat also contains gluten, a protein that cannot be digested by people with gluten intolerance or celiac disease. Because the protein cannot be broken down, the body attacks it as an allergen, causing gas, bloating, and cramping. While not all grains are equal (and some are alkaline forming, such as amaranth, millet, quinoa, and wild rice), the bulk of grains consumed by Americans today are in the form of products made with refined white flour or corn. Refined grains are also devoid of valuable B vitamins and fiber and are considered high-glycemic foods, which can cause spikes in blood sugar, triggering your body to store fat.

Sodium The 2015–2020 Dietary Guidelines for Americans recommend Americans consume less than 2,300 milligrams of sodium per day. Nearly everyone can benefit from a lower sodium intake due to its negative impact on heart health. Sodium, like sugar, can be sneaky, showing up in a vast majority of the foods we eat every day, even if we never pick up a saltshaker. Because of its acid-forming nature, choose fresh and unprocessed foods to keep your sodium intake in check.

Alkaline Foods to Enjoy

Fortunately there is no shortage of alkalizing foods that will feed your body with a bounty of vitamins, minerals, phytochemicals, and antioxidants, adding vitality and improving your health. Use the following list to learn about the health benefits of the foods to include in your diet. Focus on what you can *add*, rather than on what you need to reduce or eliminate. This subtle shift in thinking can make all the difference for you, removing stress, anxiety, and judgment. Get the good stuff in first, and you may find there isn't much room left for the unhealthy stuff.

Leafy greens Leafy green vegetables are some of the most nutritious foods you can eat, and whether you sneak them in to a smoothie or serve them in a salad, they are alkalizing and high in nutrients and phyto-chemicals. While all greens are nutritious, some of the top picks for health include kale, spinach, Swiss chard, turnip greens, arugula, and mustard greens. Nutritional powerhouses, greens are high in fiber, low in calories, and contain ample amounts of bone health–promoting calcium and vita-min K. As an added bonus, greens are rich in vitamins A and C, the alkalizing mineral potassium, and several important phyto-chemicals including lutein and zeaxanthin. Studies suggest that the carotenoids and phytochemicals found in leafy greens may protect against cataracts and certain types of cancer, lower the risk of type 2 diabetes, and be useful for weight management. Go crazy with your greens and eat them often.

Beans and lentils Beans and legumes are powerhouses of nutrition, and packed inside each bean is heart-healthy plant protein, fiber, B vitamins, iron, potassium, and little to no fat or sodium. Beans have been shown to lower the risk of heart disease and cancer, due in part to the various phytochemicals present. Beans can also lower cholesterol because they provide the body with soluble fiber, the same fiber that provides satiety, while keeping blood sugar levels steady. While some choices within this group are slightly acidic, they are far less acidifying than animal sources of protein. Some of your best bets include kidney beans (PRAL -0.5), black beans (-2.2), pigeon peas (-3.9), lima beans (-3.7), and green and yellow spilt peas (-1.0).

Nuts and seeds For many people, some of their favorite nuts are considered slightly to moderately acid forming, including walnuts, hazelnuts, peanuts, and pecans. However, there are still plenty of other varieties of nuts and seeds you can enjoy that have an alkalizing effect in the body. Chestnuts (-8.2) are ranked as the most alkaline-forming nut, due in part to their high water content, followed by almonds, which are ranked second on the alkaline scale. Nuts, even ones that are slightly acid forming, contain healthy fats, fiber, and essential vitamins and minerals, including magnesium, zinc, and vitamin E. Seeds you can enjoy on your alkaline diet include omega-3- and fiber-rich chia, hemp, and flax and vitamin E–rich sesame and sunflower. Including nuts as part of a healthy diet can benefit heart health, add key nutrients, and aid in weight management by boosting satiety.

Tubers As you work toward decreasing the grains in your diet, you may be left asking what you can eat instead to fill this void. The answer is tubers! Tubers are a group of plants that develop starchy roots and are ancient food sources prized for their amaz-ing nutritional benefits. Considered complex carbohydrates, tubers provide the body with blood sugar–stabilizing slow-burn-ing energy. High in fiber, phytochemicals, vitamins A and C, the minerals potassium and magnesium, and antioxidants, tubers can help guard against heart disease, keep your bones healthy, and lower your risk for certain types of cancer. Tubers are a great low-calorie option to use in place of other grain-based starchy carbs. Some best bets include sweet potatoes, yams, and cassava.

Crucifers You really can't find a more nutritious group of foods than the crucifers. In terms of nutrients, their stats are off the charts with high levels of vitamins A and C, carotenoids, folic acid, and fiber. Kale and collards, while leafy greens, are technically cruciferous vegetables and contain more bone health–promoting vitamin K than any other vegetable. The impressive phytochemical content of this vegetable group has been shown to lower the risk for certain types of cancer, including prostate, colorectal, lung, and breast. Low in calories and considered alkaline-forming, to reap all of their disease-protection benefits, aim for 1 to 2 cups per day. There are so many to choose from, so go for variety and try broccoli, Brussels sprouts, cabbage, collard greens, kale, bok choy, and cauliflower.

Squashes Squash is a broad term that encompasses a number of different types of vegetables, including pumpkin and summer squashes such as zucchini and crookneck, along with numerous winter varieties including acorn, Hubbard, butternut, and cushaw. Squash is extremely versatile and can be used in salads or stir-fries or julienned and used as a substitute for noodles. The impressive health benefits of squash include a high amount of vitamin A as well as ample amounts of vitamins C, E, and B and the minerals magnesium, potassium, calcium, and iron. Including squash in your diet can keep your heart healthy by adding potassium; lower inflammation levels by providing the phytochemicals lutein, zeaxanthin, and beta-carotene; and protect against certain types of cancers by adding vitamin A and carotenoids.

Nightshades Members of the *Solanaceae,* common nightshades include white potatoes, eggplant, tomatoes, sweet bell peppers, hot chile peppers, and spices made from peppers including paprika, red pepper flakes, and cayenne pepper. While a fairly small list, this group of vegetables boasts a number of important health benefits. Tomatoes are a rich source of the phytochemical lycopene, which can lower the risk of prostate cancer, while a compound in peppers, capsaicin, acts as a powerful anti-inflammatory in the body. All of these foods are high in the antioxidant vitamin C, fiber, and important minerals including heart-healthy potassium and magnesium.

Living Alkaline

Your boyfriend offers you a bowl of his butter-soaked fettuccine Alfredo. Your best friend hands you a plate with a gargantuan slice of pecan pie topped with a scoop of vanilla ice cream. Your boss sends you out of town for a conference. It's tough to eat clean and stick to a healthy eating plan when those around you are indulging or in situations where you may not have much control over your choices. But don't stress.

The following tips will help you stay on track without alienating the not-so-healthy eaters in your life and help you navigate life's other challenging food situations.

Celebrations at work Food at work is inevitable, so rather than stress about it or let it derail you, decide in advance how you will deal with temptation. One strategy is to enlist a support group of like-minded coworkers who are also eating clean. Together you can politely decline, or better yet contribute a healthy alternative such as a fruit and vegetable platter. Keep healthy snacks in your desk and office refrigerator so you can eat something healthy while others indulge. Examples include kale chips, celery sticks with almond butter, whole almonds, apples, vegetable soups, hummus, and sliced vegetables.

Business lunch or dinner Remember that you make your own choices no matter what others are doing, and you have the freedom to choose what you eat and drink. Almost all restaurants have some type of salad and vegetable on the menu, and most are willing to accommodate special diets. If the menu has a vegetable soup, order that in addition to a salad and side vegetable and make protein a side dish. Many people don't want to appear to be "high maintenance" in work situations; however, you can politely make some healthy boundaries for yourself and take control of what you can. Do keep perspective and the 80/20 Rule in mind. If your choices are less than ideal and your meal

comes in around 20/80, shoot for 90/10 the rest of the day.

Traveling Sticking to your nutritional plan can be tough when you are away from home for extended periods of time, but it can be done by being proactive. Take time to research restaurants and supermarkets ahead of time. Pack healthy snacks that won't spoil easily, like almonds and apples. If you are traveling by car, take a cooler packed with vegetables, fruits, seeds, avocados, and tubers. If you are staying at a hotel, call ahead and request a refrigerator and microwave. You can stick to the Alkaline Diet while traveling. All it takes is a bit of research, planning, and commitment.

Holidays Holidays can be tough on the waistline even when you aren't following a special diet. The best strategy is to be proactive and prepare alkaline-friendly dishes to share at holiday gatherings. Remember that it's okay to allow a few treats; just practice portion control and fill the majority of your plate with healthy foods.

Sabotage from a spouse or partner If your spouse or partner isn't on board with your Alkaline Diet, he or she may feel threatened, causing a negative reaction. To prevent this from happening, be certain to ask for their support *before* you embark on the Alkaline Diet. Let them know that preparing healthier versions of the family's favorite foods is a great way for you to show your love. Ask for their help in choosing recipes, and get them involved in planning meals.

WHO DECIDES?

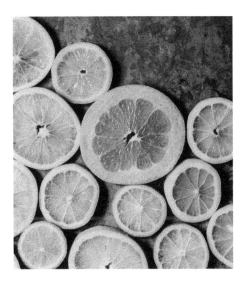

D o an Internet search for "acid-alkaline food chart," and you'll find there is no shortage of results. The problem is they all seem to be different. How can a food be classified as acidic on one chart and alkaline on another? Isn't that like saying red is blue and blue is red? Can a food be both acidic and alkaline? The short answer is yes, and that is because some lists define foods by their pH in whole physical form before they are eaten. In this case, a lemon would be acidic and milk and chicken alkaline. This seems rationale and intuitive. However, this method does not take into account the impact of the food on the body after it is digested and metabolized. This is where the PRAL score comes into play. The PRAL (potential renal acid load) score, developed by researchers Remer and Manz, is a scientific way to measure the acid load of any food based on the protein, phosphorus, potassium, magnesium, and calcium content of a 100 gram serving. Negative numbers (–) are good and indicate the potential alkalinity being contributed by a base-forming food. Positive numbers (+) indicate the potential acidity being contributed by an acid-forming food. You will still find inconsistencies even with PRAL numbers as research evolves, so use the scores as a general guide for filling your plate with nutritious foods, and don't stress or micromanage your food choices.

Weekends The structure of a weekday routine makes it easier to stick to a healthy eating plan, but for whatever reason the weekends throw a wrench into things. There can be room for splurges, but keep your healthy goals in the back of your mind when making choices. Stay focused and consistent, and try to continue with regular healthy meals and exercise. If desired, allow yourself a splurge here and there, but keep portions in check. Always start with a healthy breakfast, keep things simple, and stick to the basics including lean protein, healthy fats, and lots of fruits and vegetables so that you will feel full longer and feel satisfied with small splurges.

Managing hunger Allowing yourself to get overly hungry is one of the quickest ways to get off track with your Alkaline Diet. Regularize your eating with a set plan of meals and snacks. Some people do well with no snacks and some with a snack after each meal. While you should let physical hunger be your guide, often stress overrides our natural cues, leading us to ignore our need for nourishment. Take time once a week to plan your meals and snacks for the week, and keep your body fueled throughout the day.

Happy hour Alcoholic drinks can be calorie bombs, and they are also highly acidic in the body. Know your options and choose wisely: Seltzer water is just plain water with some bubbles added, so it's zero calories. Tonic water, on the other hand, has 120 calories—all from sugar. Volunteer to be the designated driver, and your friends will surely thank you and not question your drink choices.

What About Exercise?

Physical activity is another essential component for decreasing your risk for chronic disease, maintaining a healthy weight, and managing stress. The *2008 Physical Activity Guidelines for Americans* provide evidence-based guidance for Americans aged 6 and older for appropriate levels and types of activity. A summary of those recommendations follows.

Key Guidelines for Children and Adolescents

- Children and adolescents should do 60 minutes or more of physical activity daily.

- Most of the 60 minutes a day should be either moderate- or vigorous-intensity aerobic physical activity, and vigorous activity should be included at least 3 days a week.

- As part of their daily 60 minutes of activity, children and adolescents should include muscle-strengthening and bone-strengthening activities at least 3 days a week.

Key Guidelines for Adults

- For substantial health benefits, adults should do at least 150 minutes a week of moderate-intensity or 75 minutes a week of vigorous-intensity exercise, or an equivalent combination of the two. Ideally, aerobic exercise should be performed in bouts of at least 10 minutes.

- For more extensive health benefits, adults should increase their aerobic physical activity to 300 minutes a week of moderate-intensity or 150 minutes a week of vigorous-intensity activity.

- Adults should also do muscle-strengthening activities involving all major muscle groups two or more days a week.

Key Guidelines for Older Adults

- When older adults cannot do 150 minutes of moderate-intensity activity per week because of chronic conditions, they should be as physically active as their abilities and conditions allow.

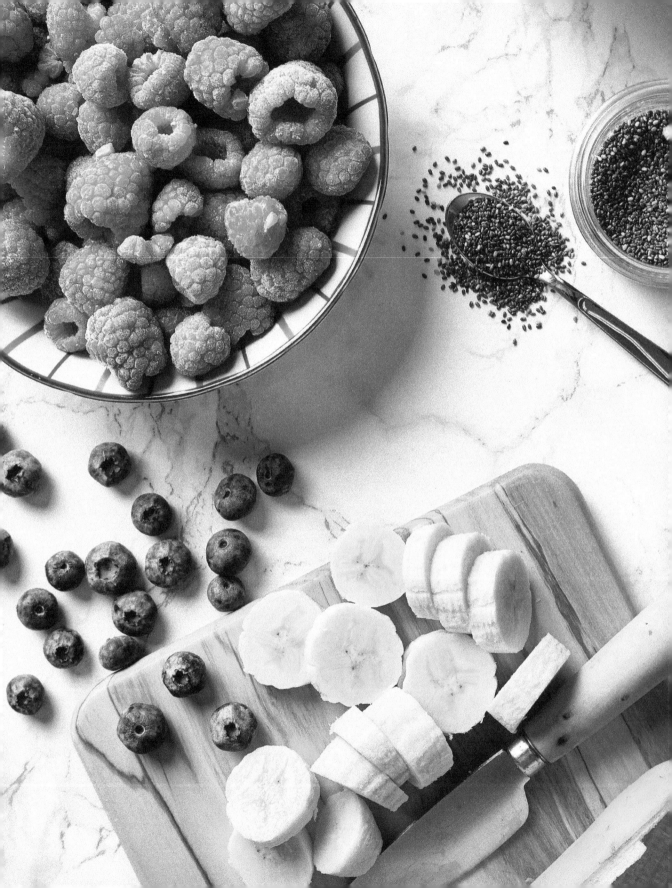

CHAPTER TWO

30-Day Meal Plan

Now that you have decided to try the Alkaline Diet, where do you start? Transitioning to an alkaline lifestyle may seem overwhelming at first, but often the *idea* of change is more daunting than actually doing it. Can you ease into the alkaline lifestyle? Of course you can. However, it is typically best to give it your gusto from the get-go. And, just like most things in life, the will to succeed means nothing without the will to prepare.

It is often helpful to time your start when you know you can focus on your diet without additional challenges such as travel or social obligations. Choose a time when your life is relatively calm, you have a little free time to prepare healthy meals, and your routine is unlikely to change much in the coming few months. If you have an extra vacation day, consider taking a three-day weekend to set yourself up for success.

The first thing you will want to do is review the menus and recipes in this book and become familiar with the ingredients used, the steps involved, and the equipment needed. The good news is that you will be using fresh, whole foods and preparing meals that are quick and uncomplicated. Choose a day for menu planning, shopping, and preparation. You may find it works best to shop once a week, twice a week, or every other day depending on your schedule. Try using Sunday afternoons to prep veggies, sauces, and snacks in advance so they are ready to grab-n-go during the week.

When transitioning to an Alkaline Diet, remember not to make too many changes at once. Just take it day-by-day, meal-by-meal, and keep things simple. In fact, the simpler your meals, the better they are for you. Now let's get started with week one.

CURBING CRAVINGS

Here are some tips for dealing with cravings for highly acid-forming items such as pepperoni pizza, coffee, and alcoholic drinks.

CHECK YOUR HYDRATION

Hunger is often mistaken for thirst. Check your hydration, and aim to drink water throughout the day.

ADDRESS THE EMOTIONAL COMPONENT OF YOUR FOOD CRAVINGS

Are you physically hungry, or is it psychological hunger? Are you actually tired, sad, stressed, bored, lonely, or angry? Check in with yourself, and get a mood boost from somewhere else: Splurge on a massage, go somewhere new and interesting, or plan a surprise for someone else.

GET UP AND MOVE

A tried-and-true trick for kicking cravings to the curb is to get up and get active! Tell yourself you will postpone eating whatever your craving is until you get back from your workout. Then go get sweaty: Take a brisk walk, go to the gym, or go for a run. While you are working out, you'll release those feel-good endorphins, and once you are feeling good, you will want to feed your body with nutritious foods.

EAT REGULARLY

Prevent cravings by eating regularly and aiming for a balance of nutrients at each meal and snack. Visualize your plate, and fill half with veggies/fruits, one-quarter with protein, and one-quarter with high-fiber complex carbs. Cravings for fat, salt, and sugar may mean your meals are out of balance.

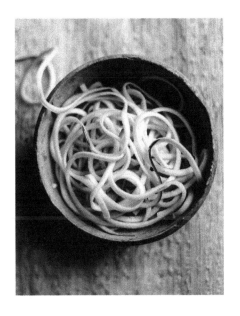

REPLACE IT

Make an alkaline replacement of the food you are craving. Try spiralizing zucchini as a replacement for pasta or replacing butter on bread with avocado.

REMOVE "IT" OR YOURSELF

Avoid temptation in the first place by removing junk food and processed foods from your pantry. Place a fruit bowl on your kitchen counter within plain view and replace ice cream with blended frozen bananas.

ADD NATURAL FLAVORS

Counter cravings for sugar, fat, and salt by using fresh herbs and spices to boost flavor. Roast your veggies to bring out their natural sweetness.

WAIT IT OUT

Research shows that you can wait out cravings by distracting yourself. Any random activity will work; just focus on something else for at least 10 minutes to get the craving out of your head. Write down your health goals, read a book, do some cleaning, or call a friend.

Week One

1

The fundamental key to success with any lifestyle modification is removal, elimination, and avoidance of the "agents" opposing your desired lifestyle. In other words, you need to eliminate the Standard American Diet foods that promise to thwart you at every turn. To do this, summon up your courage and purge your kitchen of junk food in a dramatic blaze of glory so you'll stick to your convictions. If a food isn't conducive to your goals, why keep it? Be prepared for some pushback from your inner self with defensive, self-justifying excuses: I hate wasting food; it was on sale; my kid/husband/wife/roommate likes these; it's for special occasions (like this Thursday, when I'll have a bad day at work). If it won't help you reach your goals, you don't need it. A kitchen makeover gets rid of the non-nutritious foods or foods that trigger poor decisions and replaces them with a bounty of health-promoting foods to help you stay on track.

The first thing you need to do is head into the kitchen and get a large garbage bag or some boxes. If the food is nonperishable, donate it to a local food bank or soup kitchen. The best way to figure out whether you should keep a food is to ask yourself a few questions:

- Does this food come in a bag, box, or plastic package?

- Does it have more than a couple of ingredients on the label?

- Can you pronounce the ingredients?

- Is this food perishable? In general, healthy foods will spoil quickly.

Once you have finished purging, a good way to quickly restock is to create a list of your favorite four or five vegetables, fruits, nuts/seeds, lean proteins, whole grains, and tubers. Use your list and the suggested weekly menu to write a grocery list and then go shopping. Try to shop for seasonal, organic, and local items whenever possible.

Stocking a healthy kitchen looks less daunting when you lay it out like that, and once you have everything dialed in and you're eating whole foods, you won't miss the other stuff.

1

MONDAY

Breakfast Strawberry and Chia Seed Overnight Oats Parfait

Lunch Beefless "Beef" Stew

Dinner Cheesy Scallop Potato and Onion Bake

Snacks Parsley and Tahini Hummus with Tarragon Crackers

TUESDAY

Breakfast Hemp Seed and Banana Green Smoothie

Lunch Cashew-Broccoli Salad with Spicy Cashew Dressing

Dinner Lentil and Sweet Potato Taco Wraps

Snacks Cheesy Baked Kale Chips; Chewy Nut and Seed Bars

WEDNESDAY

Breakfast Pumpkin Seed–Protein Breakfast Balls

Lunch Mushroom-Lentil Salad with Lime-Tahini Dressing

Dinner Roasted Cauliflower Wraps with Mango-Habanero Sauce

Snacks Blueberry-Banana "Ice Cream"; Paprika-Garlic Almonds

THURSDAY

Breakfast Carrot and Hemp Seed Muffins

Lunch Wild Rice and Mushroom-Miso Soup

Dinner Sweet Potato Slices with Roasted Red Pepper and Artichoke Spread

Snacks Peach and Kale Protein Smoothie; Cheesy Broccoli Bites

FRIDAY

Breakfast Frozen Banana–Protein Breakfast Bowl

Lunch Red Lentil Penne Pasta Salad with Sautéed Vegetables

Dinner Spicy Eggplant Stir-Fry

Snacks Oregano and Garlic Breadsticks; Cashew Butter Fudge

SATURDAY

Breakfast Vanilla Bean and Cinnamon Granola

Lunch Creamy Lentil and Potato Stew

Dinner Nori Veggie Rolls with Avocado-Jalapeño Spread

Snacks Peach and Kale Protein Smoothie Parsley; Parsley and Tahini Hummus

SUNDAY

Breakfast Sweet Potato and Kale Breakfast Hash

Lunch Roasted Carrot and Onion Salad with Creamy Cashew-Miso Dressing

Dinner Lentil and Cucumber Pasta Bowl

Snacks Lemon and Garlic Cashew Cream-Stuffed Mushrooms; Apple Pie Crumble

Week Two

2

Congratulations on making it to week two of your Alkaline Diet! The human body is an amazing machine, but exactly what you'll experience when you reduce acid-forming foods in your diet will depend on how Westernized your diet was before you started. People on the high end of the Standard American Diet spectrum may show addict-like withdrawal symptoms in the first few days or week, including anxiety, headaches, restlessness, and even depression. When cravings strike, and they will, use the tips in the sidebar Curbing Cravings (page 30) to wrestle them back into their cage.

One of the first changes you will notice is improved digestion, from a decrease in gas and bloating to an increase in healthy bowel movements. An Alkaline Diet is high in fiber and natural pre- and probiotics that help populate the good bacteria in your intestines.

Once you start flushing out toxins, your skin may actually look worse before it looks better, but within two weeks you should see improvements.

And while your disposition may not improve immediately due to withdrawal symptoms from caffeine and sugar, by day three or four, the "brain fog" will begin to lift and you can expect an increase in mental clarity, memory, concentration, and focus. There's no mistaking that eliminating caffeine and sugar can be a mood buster, but stick with it and by week two you will see improvements in sleep, energy, and frame of mind.

As you continue your transition, you can expect to feel healthier and more energetic and may even lose a few pounds. You might be surprised how full you feel and how satisfying and satiating real foods are. You may not be able to describe it, but you will just "feel better."

2

MONDAY

Breakfast Lemon-Ginger Green Smoothie

Lunch Peach Salsa Salad with Sweet Tahini Dressing

Dinner Stuffed Sweet Potato with Broccoli-Basil Pesto

Snacks Paprika-Garlic Almonds; Parsley and Tahini Hummus

TUESDAY

Breakfast Oatmeal Porridge with Mango-Chia Fruit Jam

Lunch Roasted Carrot and Leek Soup

Dinner Lentil and Cucumber Pasta Bowl

Snacks Oregano and Garlic Breadsticks; Chewy Nut and Seed Bars

WEDNESDAY

Breakfast Mixed Berry–Chia Seed Pudding

Lunch Warm Asparagus Salad with Lemon-Asparagus Dressing

Dinner Cheesy Scallop Potato and Onion Bake

Snacks Peach and Kale Protein Smoothie; Cinnamon Cashews

THURSDAY

Breakfast Avocado–Sweet Potato "Toast"

Lunch Creamy Lentil and Potato Stew

Dinner Veggie-Stuffed Portobello Mushrooms

Snacks Raspberry-Lime Smoothie; Cheesy Baked Kale Chips

FRIDAY

Breakfast No-Bake Granola Bars

Lunch Fresh Herb Potato Salad

Dinner Fresh Veggie Pizza with Tahini-Beet Spread

Snacks Lemon and Garlic Cashew Cream–Stuffed Mushrooms; Hemp Seed and Banana Green Smoothie

SATURDAY

Breakfast Raspberry-Avocado Smoothie Bowl

Lunch Roasted Beet–Kale Salad with Lemon-Garlic Vinaigrette

Dinner Spicy Cilantro-Lentil "Burgers"

Snacks Chipotle-Jicama Fries with Scallion Dip; Pear Nachos with Sweetened Almond Butter Drizzle

SUNDAY

Breakfast Pineapple and Coconut Oatmeal Bowl

Lunch Creamy Green Olive Pasta Salad

Dinner Zucchini and Kale Pesto Spaghetti Squash

Snacks Cashew Butter Fudge; Peach and Kale Protein Smoothie

Week Three

3

By this time you should find that your taste buds have recalibrated and eating junk is not as enjoyable as you remember. Once you eat clean, the taste of processed foods and all of the salt, sugar, and fat will be overwhelming—another reminder of how food is engineered to be addictive and a reminder of the many reasons to put your health first and stick to your alkaline eating plan.

By about week three along your journey, you will find yourself discovering new favorite foods and developing new habits. Instead of shopping the inside aisles of the grocery store, you will be loading your cart with fresh foods located in the perimeter. Maybe now you spend a Sunday afternoon making big pots of beans and prepping fruits, vegetables, and homemade sauces and snacks for the week ahead.

Instead of blindly picking up packaged food, you will start reading labels on everything you buy. The shock of finding so many unnecessary processed ingredients will make you an impulsive ingredient reader. Sugar in deli meat and marinara sauce? Salt in meat, cereals, breads, canned beans, and soups? It's amazing how quickly the amounts add up and equally amazing how quickly you can do your heart a favor by preparing your own homemade versions. Preparing foods yourself means you have so much more control over what you are eating. And while prepping takes more time initially, once you find the habits that work for you, it'll start becoming a natural part of your routine.

MONDAY

Breakfast Blueberry Green Smoothie

Lunch Pineapple Salad with Lime Vinaigrette

Dinner Wild Rice and Broccoli Bowl with Roasted Garlic Sauce

Snacks Cheesy Baked Kale Chips; Parsley and Tahini Hummus

TUESDAY

Breakfast Sesame and Hemp Seed Breakfast Cookies

Lunch Coconut, Cilantro, and Jalapeño Soup

Dinner Creamy Artichoke and Basil Red Lentil Penne Pasta

Snacks Paprika-Garlic Almonds; Peach and Kale Protein Smoothie

WEDNESDAY

Breakfast Raspberry-Lime Smoothie

Lunch Mushroom-Lentil Salad with Lime-Tahini Dressing

Dinner Lentil and Cucumber Pasta Bowl

Snacks Oregano and Garlic Breadsticks; Blueberry-Banana "Ice Cream"

THURSDAY

Breakfast Frozen Banana–Protein Breakfast Bowl

Lunch Spicy Chilled Red Pepper Soup

Dinner Cheesy Scallop Potato and Onion Bake

Snacks Paprika-Garlic Almonds; Chewy Nut and Seed Bars

FRIDAY

Breakfast Pumpkin Seed–Protein Breakfast Balls

Lunch Creamy Lentil and Potato Stew

Dinner Fresh Veggie Pizza with Tahini-Beet Spread

Snacks Cheesy Broccoli Bites; Cinnamon Cashews

SATURDAY

Breakfast Blackberry and Avocado Smoothie

Lunch Sweet Potato Slices with Roasted Red Pepper and Artichoke Spread

Dinner Roasted Cauliflower Wraps with Mango-Habanero Sauce

Snacks Cashew Butter Fudge; Flourless Pumpkin Seed Cookies

SUNDAY

Breakfast Fresh Fruit with Vanilla-Cashew Cream

Lunch Roasted Garlic and Cauliflower Soup

Dinner Warm Sweet Potato Salad with Jalapeño-Cilantro Dressing

Snacks No-Bake Granola Bars; Thumbprint Cookies with Blueberry–Chia Seed Jam

3

Week Four

4

Congratulations on reaching week four of your Alkaline Diet! Research shows that it takes about 30 days to form a new habit, so you should find yourself doing things more automatically at this point, like reading ingredient lists on everything you buy, reaching for herbal tea instead of coffee, and adding kale to your smoothies like a champ. Think about improving your eating habits as consisting of a number of small, manageable steps, like adding a salad to your diet once a day. You start by making one small, permanent change that you can live with until it becomes habit, and then you pick another small change to tackle.

After a month of clean alkaline eating, some health benefits you may experience include better blood sugar control, normalized blood pressure, increased energy, and better sleep. Perhaps your clothes are a tad looser and your mind a bit clearer. Without processed foods overriding your body's natural hunger and fullness cues, you may find you snack less, and when you do snack, what you consume is better for you, like fruits, vegetables, and nuts.

Looking ahead, educate yourself as much as you can about what foods to avoid and substitutions you can make. Make meal planning a must, and use time-saving appliances such as slow cookers for batch cooking and freezing. And don't forget to make room for related goals like exercise. A brisk morning walk can wake you up and energize you better than any caffeinated beverage.

Finally, be around other like-minded people. It can be hard to follow an Alkaline Diet when all of your friends, family, and coworkers are eating a typical Standard American Diet. Spending time with other people who share your goals will inspire you to stay on track.

As you continue your journey toward a fully alkaline lifestyle, continue to reflect on your habits, both good and bad, replace unhealthy habits with healthy ones, and reinforce your new, healthier eating habits. Most of all, have fun discovering new foods and take it one food, one meal, one day at a time.

MONDAY

Breakfast Hemp Seed and Banana Green Smoothie

Lunch Roasted Carrot and Onion Salad with Creamy Cashew-Miso Dressing

Dinner Spicy Eggplant Stir-Fry

Snacks Tarragon Crackers; Lemon and Garlic Cashew Cream–Stuffed Mushrooms

TUESDAY

Breakfast Avocado–Sweet Potato "Toast"

Lunch Roasted Garlic and Cauliflower Soup

Dinner Lentil and Sweet Potato Taco Wraps

Snacks Raspberry-Lime Smoothie; Cinnamon Cashews

WEDNESDAY

Breakfast Watermelon-Cherry Smoothie

Lunch Mushroom-Lentil Salad with Lime-Tahini Dressing

Dinner Beefless "Beef" Stew

Snacks Cheesy Broccoli Bites; Pear Nachos with Sweetened Almond Butter Drizzle

THURSDAY

Breakfast Strawberry and Chia Seed Overnight Oats Parfait

Lunch Broccoli and Potato Soup

Dinner Nori Veggie Rolls with Avocado-Jalapeño Spread

Snacks Baked Avocado Fries; Paprika-Garlic Almonds

FRIDAY

Breakfast Sesame and Hemp Seed Breakfast Cookies

Lunch Blueberry and Fennel Salad with Roasted Garlic and Miso Dressing

Dinner Creamy Lentil and Potato Stew

Snacks Cheesy Baked Kale Chips; Apple Pie Crumble

SATURDAY

Breakfast Carrot and Hemp Seed Muffins

Lunch Watermelon-Basil Salad with Basil Vinaigrette

Dinner Stuffed Sweet Potato with Broccoli-Basil Pesto

Snacks Blueberry and Kiwi Hemp Seed Smoothie; Lemon and Garlic Cashew Cream–Stuffed Mushrooms

SUNDAY

Breakfast Blueberry and Chia Seed Cobbler

Lunch Red Lentil Penne Pasta Salad with Sautéed Vegetables

Dinner Cheesy Scallop Potato and Onion Bake

Snacks Peach and Kale Protein Smoothie; Vanilla Bean and Coconut Truffles

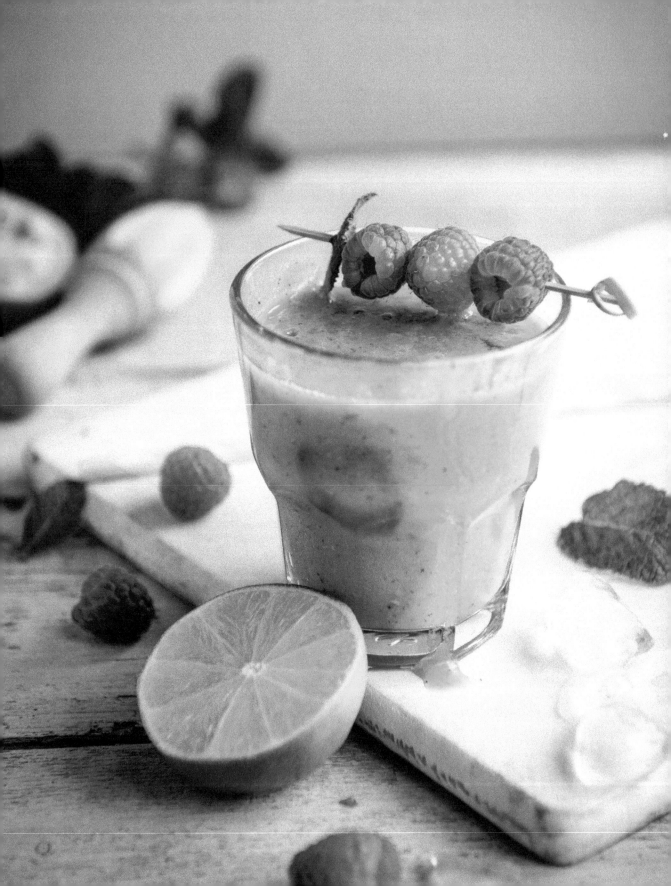

CHAPTER THREE

Smoothies Galore

Mango and Kiwi Smoothie

Serves 1 or 2
Prep: 5 minutes

QUICK & EASY

This tropical smoothie is naturally sweetened with mango and kiwi. Cashews give it a slightly creamy texture, but you could leave them out if you prefer or are nut-free. Although the ice cubes are optional, they transform the smoothie into a frosty treat to start your mornings. Want to give it an extra nutritional boost? Garnish with unsweetened shredded coconut flakes, hemp seeds, or chia seeds.

1½ cups coconut milk (boxed)

½ cup chopped mango

1 kiwi, peeled and chopped

¼ cup raw cashews

5 to 7 ice cubes (optional)

In a high-speed blender, blend to combine the coconut milk, mango, kiwi, cashews, and ice (if using) until smooth.

Pour into 1 large or 2 small glasses and enjoy.

TIP For a fun summertime treat, use the mixture to make frozen ice pop treats in your favorite ice pop molds—just omit the ice cubes! Vitamix is a great high-speed blender when you want your smoothie completely smooth.

Blueberry and Kiwi Hemp Seed Smoothie

WEEK 4
Serves 1 or 2
Prep: 5 minutes

QUICK & EASY

Not only does this smoothie contain high-alkaline kiwi and high-antioxidant blueberries, it also gets a boost of plant-based protein (10.6 grams in a 2-tablespoon serving) from hemp seeds. If you use fresh blueberries, you may want to add some ice cubes to get a lovely frosty texture. You can even add extra hemp seeds on top to garnish!

1½ cups almond milk

1 kiwi, peeled and chopped

1 cup fresh or frozen blueberries

2 tablespoons hemp seeds

5 to 7 ice cubes (optional)

In a blender, blend to combine the almond milk, kiwi, blueberries, hemp seeds, and ice (if using) until smooth.

Pour into 1 large or 2 small glasses and enjoy.

TIP Make this a nut-free recipe by substituting the almond milk with coconut milk.

Watermelon-Cherry Smoothie

WEEK 4
Serves 1 or 2
Prep: 5 minutes

`QUICK & EASY` `NUT-FREE`

This light and refreshing smoothie is made with super-hydrating watermelon and anti-inflammatory cherries for the perfect summer beverage. The recipe calls for dark sweet cherries, but you could use your favorite variety. If cherries aren't in season, you can use frozen cherries.

2 cups cubed watermelon
10 pitted dark sweet cherries
1 cup coconut milk (boxed)
1 tablespoon brown rice syrup
1 tablespoon freshly squeezed lime juice
5 to 7 ice cubes (optional)

In a blender, blend to combine the watermelon, cherries, coconut milk, brown rice syrup, lime juice, and ice (if using) until smooth.

Pour into 1 large or 2 small glasses and enjoy.

TIP If you prefer your smoothie a little sweeter, substitute the brown rice syrup with half a banana.

Blackberry and Avocado Smoothie

WEEK 3
Serves 1 or 2
Prep: 5 minutes

`QUICK & EASY` `NUT-FREE`

Adding avocado to a smoothie gives it a thick, creamy texture and healthy fat. And don't worry: your smoothie won't taste like avocado. Avocados are also an excellent source of vitamin E, and 1 cup provides 24 percent of your daily value of vitamin C. The banana adds just the right hint of sweetness.

1½ cups coconut milk
1 cup blackberries
½ avocado, roughly chopped
½ banana, roughly chopped

In a blender, blend to combine the coconut milk, blackberries, avocado, and banana until creamy and smooth.

Pour into 1 large or 2 small glasses and enjoy.

TIP You can substitute the blackberries with another alkaline fruit like blueberries, strawberries, or raspberries.

Avocado and Kale Smoothie

Serves 1 or 2
Prep: 5 minutes

QUICK & EASY

This green smoothie is packed with lots of nutrients like balanced, healthy omega fatty acids from the hemp seeds, healthy fat and fiber from the avocado, and vitamins K and A from the kale. It's naturally sweetened with half a banana, so it's not overly sweet, but feel free to use the whole banana if you prefer your smoothie a little sweeter. The avocado is added not only for its nutritional benefits, but because it will give the smoothie a thicker and creamier texture. Any variety of kale will work—just make sure you stem it before adding it to your blender.

1½ cups almond milk

2 kale stalks, stemmed

½ avocado, roughly chopped

½ banana, roughly chopped

1 tablespoon hemp seeds

In a blender, blend to combine the almond milk, kale, avocado, banana, and hemp seeds until creamy and smooth.

Pour into 1 large or 2 small glasses and enjoy.

TIP Substitute the almond milk with coconut milk for a nut-free version.

Hemp Seed and Banana Green Smoothie

WEEKS 1, 2 & 3
Serves 1 or 2
Prep: 5 minutes

QUICK & EASY

Hemp seeds and almond butter are amazing plant-based proteins, adding about 17 grams of protein to the smoothie, and red chard is an amazing source of vitamins K, A, and C. Add the ice cubes if you like your smoothies cool and icy.

1½ cups coconut milk (boxed)

½ to 1 banana, roughly chopped

½ cup chopped rainbow or red chard

2 tablespoons almond butter

2 tablespoons hemp seeds

5 to 7 ice cubes (optional)

In a blender, blend to combine the coconut milk, banana, chard, almond butter, hemp seeds, and ice (if using) until creamy and smooth.

Pour into 1 large or 2 small glasses and enjoy.

TIP Substitute the chard with kale.

Blueberry Green Smoothie

WEEK 3
Serves 1 or 2
Prep: 5 minutes

`QUICK & EASY` `NUT-FREE`

This rich, smooth beverage is just the ticket to starting your morning well. The cucumbers and blueberries are an excellent source of antioxidants, and both are anti-inflammatory. If you use fresh blueberries, you may want to add the ice cubes to make it nice and cool.

1½ cups coconut milk (boxed)

1 avocado, roughly chopped

1 cucumber, peeled and roughly chopped

½ to 1 banana, roughly chopped

1 cup fresh or frozen blueberries

5 to 7 ice cubes (optional)

In a blender, blend to combine the coconut milk, avocado, cucumber, banana, blueberries, and ice (if using) until creamy and smooth.

Pour into 1 large or 2 small glasses and enjoy.

TIP Increase the greens in this smoothie by adding 1 stemmed kale leaf.

Peach and Kale Protein Smoothie

WEEKS 1, 2 & 4
Serves 1 or 2
Prep: 5 minutes

`QUICK & EASY` `NUT-FREE`

Commercial protein powders are usually made with highly processed, unnecessary ingredients. A complete protein with 19 grams of protein in one serving, pumpkin protein powder, made from 100 percent organic pumpkin seeds, is an easy and healthy way to add quality plant-based protein to your smoothies, desserts, and other snacks.

1½ cups coconut milk (boxed)

2 romaine lettuce leaves

1 kale stalk, stemmed

1 peach, roughly chopped

½ to 1 banana, roughly chopped

5 tablespoons pumpkin protein powder

5 to 7 ice cubes (optional)

In a blender, blend to combine the coconut milk, lettuce, kale, peach, banana, pumpkin protein powder, and ice (if using) until smooth.

Pour into 1 large or 2 small glasses and enjoy.

TIP If you can't find 100 percent pumpkin protein powder, it's okay to omit it.

Lemon-Ginger Green Smoothie

WEEK 2

Serves 1 or 2
Prep: 5 minutes

QUICK & EASY   NUT-FREE

Lemon and ginger root imbue this smoothie with lots of antioxidant and anti-inflammatory goodness. Nutrient-dense greens kale and romaine lettuce give it its bright green color as well as essential vitamins K and A. Because ginger has a natural spicy (but delicious) bite, start with a small piece and add until the beverage tastes just right.

1½ cups coconut milk (boxed)

2 stalks kale, stemmed and roughly chopped

2 stalks romaine lettuce, roughly chopped

½ celery stalk, roughly chopped

1 apple, cored and roughly chopped

1 tablespoon freshly squeezed lemon juice

¼- to ½-inch piece ginger root, peeled and chopped

5 to 7 ice cubes (optional)

In a high-speed blender, blend to combine the coconut milk, kale, romaine, celery, apple, lemon juice, ginger, and ice (if using) until smooth.

Pour into 1 large or 2 small glasses and enjoy.

TIP To get the maximum benefits of lemon, use freshly squeezed as bottled lemon juice is typically pasteurized.

Raspberry-Lime Smoothie

WEEKS 2, 3 & 4

Serves 1 or 2
Prep: 5 minutes

QUICK & EASY   NUT-FREE

Berries are an excellent source of anti-oxidants, and this smoothie contains raspberries, which are one of my favorites. It's naturally sweetened with half a banana, but if you prefer your smoothie a little sweeter, go ahead and add the other half. Though you might not think immediately of pairing them, the touch of lime here really complements the raspberry and banana flavors. To make the refreshing pink color of the smoothie even more visually appealing, garnish with 1 or 2 small mint leaves.

1½ cups coconut milk (boxed)

1 cup raspberries

½ banana

1 teaspoon freshly squeezed lime juice

5 to 7 ice cubes (optional)

Fresh mint leaves, for garnish (optional)

In a blender, blend to combine the coconut milk, raspberries, banana, lime juice, and mint leaves (if using) until well combined and smooth.

Pour into 1 or 2 glasses and enjoy.

TIP Increase the nutritional profile of this smoothie by adding 2 scoops of pumpkin protein powder.

Triple Berry Protein Smoothie

Serves 1 large or 2 small
Prep: 5 minutes

QUICK & EASY NUT-FREE

Berries are an excellent source of antioxidants, and this smoothie contains three different types of berries: raspberries, blueberries, and blackberries. If you want to increase the nutritional benefits of this smoothie, you can use the smaller wild blueberries instead of the larger regular cultivated blueberries, as they contain twice the amount of antioxidants.

1½ cups coconut milk (boxed)

⅓ cup raspberries

⅓ cup blueberries

⅓ cup blackberries

3 tablespoons 100% pumpkin protein powder

In a blender, blend to combine the coconut milk, raspberries, blueberries, blackberries, and pumpkin protein powder until well combined and smooth.

TIP If you'd like a sweeter smoothie, just add ½ banana.

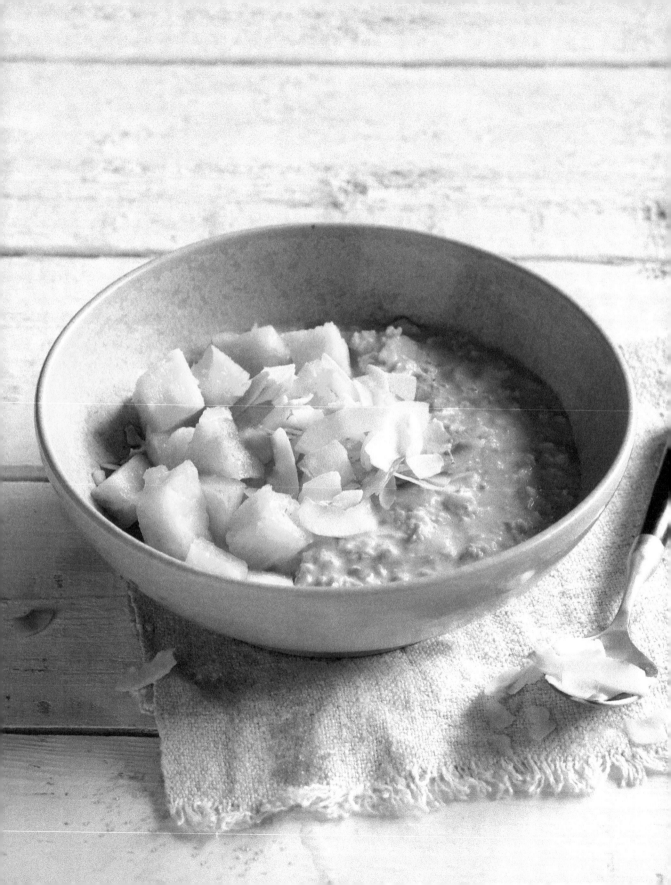

CHAPTER FOUR

Balanced Breakfasts

Strawberry and Chia Seed Overnight Oats Parfait

WEEKS 1 & 4

Serves 1 or 2

Prep: 10 minutes, plus overnight to set

Cook: None

NUT-FREE

A perfect make-ahead breakfast for those busy mornings, this delicious parfait can be made the night before to enjoy the next morning or to grab and go on your way out the door. A simple breakfast that will keep you satisfied throughout the morning, it is an excellent source of fiber and calcium from the chia seeds. You'll need to keep it covered in the refrigerator, so glass mason jars are perfect.

FOR THE STRAWBERRY MIXTURE

1 cup diced strawberries

1 teaspoon chia seeds

1 to 2 teaspoons brown rice syrup

FOR THE OAT MIXTURE

1 cup quick rolled oats

1 cup coconut milk (boxed)

1 tablespoon brown rice syrup

⅛ tablespoon vanilla bean powder

TO PREPARE THE STRAWBERRY MIXTURE

In a small bowl, stir together the strawberries, chia seeds, and brown rice syrup until well combined.

TO PREPARE THE OAT MIXTURE

In a small bowl, stir together the oats, coconut milk, brown rice syrup, and vanilla bean powder until well combined.

Place half the oat mixture in the bottom of 1 large glass mason jar or 2 small jars, and layer half of the strawberry mixture over the oat mixture. Repeat with the remaining oat and strawberry mixtures.

Cover the mason jar(s), and refrigerate overnight.

Uncover and enjoy.

TIP Substitute the strawberries with your favorite alkaline fruit like mango, pineapple, or kiwi, and feel free to use almond milk instead of coconut milk if you don't need a nut-free version.

Carrot and Hemp Seed Muffins

WEEKS 1 & 4
Makes 12 muffins
Prep: 5 minutes
Cook: 25 minutes

`QUICK & EASY`

These grain-free breakfast muffins are just as moist, and hold together as well, as muffins made with white flour and refined sugar. They are amazing right out of the oven but can also be frozen to enjoy later. Save time by making your own oat flour in advance: Just add quick rolled oats to a food processor, process until the oats turn into a flour consistency, and store in an airtight container. Hemp seeds and a subtle amount of chopped kale give these tasty muffins an extra nutritional boost.

3 tablespoons water

1 tablespoon ground flaxseed

2 cups oat flour

1 cup almond milk (boxed)

½ cup unrefined whole cane sugar, such as Sucanat

1 carrot, shredded

6 tablespoons cashew butter

2 tablespoons hemp seeds

1 tablespoon chopped lacinato kale

1 tablespoon baking powder

⅛ teaspoon vanilla bean powder

Pinch sea salt

Preheat the oven to 350°F.

To prepare a flax egg, in a small bowl, whisk together the water and flaxseed.

Transfer the flax egg to a medium bowl, and add the oat flour, almond milk, sugar, carrot, cashew butter, hemp seeds, kale, baking powder, vanilla bean powder, and salt, stirring until well combined.

Divide the mixture evenly among 12 muffin cups, bake for 20 to 25 minutes, and enjoy right away.

TIP Unrefined whole cane sugars, like Sucanat, are much less processed than regular sugar and have a higher molasses content as well. You can find Sucanat and other unrefined whole cane sugars at natural food stores or online.

Raspberry-Avocado Smoothie Bowl

WEEK 2

Serves 2
Prep: 5 minutes
Cook: None

`QUICK & EASY` `NUT-FREE`

Smoothie bowls are amazing, not only for their taste, but they also give you a chance to sit down and enjoy the same benefits of a grab-and-go smoothie, albeit in a bowl. Smoothie bowls are a little thicker than a regular smoothie, and you get to add more toppings than you would be able to in a smoothie cup.

1½ cups coconut milk (boxed)

1 cup raspberries, plus more (optional) for topping

1 avocado, roughly chopped

3 tablespoons unrefined whole cane sugar, such as Sucanat, divided

1 teaspoon chia seeds

1 teaspoon unsweetened shredded coconut

Mixed berries, for topping (optional)

In a blender, blend to combine the coconut milk, raspberries, avocado, and 2 tablespoons of sugar until smooth and creamy.

Pour the mixture into 2 serving bowls, sprinkle the extra raspberries (if using), the remaining 1 tablespoon of the sugar, and the chia seeds, shredded coconut, and mixed berries (if using) over the top, and enjoy.

TIP Smoothie bowls are customizable! Substitute the raspberries with blackberries, blueberries, or mango. You can even add or change the toppings, too—try hemp seeds, sunflower seeds, or other alkaline fruits.

Sweet Potato and Kale Breakfast Hash

WEEK 1

Serves 1 or 2
Prep: 10 minutes
Cook: 15 minutes

`QUICK & EASY` `NUT-FREE`

Sometimes a savory breakfast is in order, but that doesn't mean it has to be complicated. This breakfast dish can be ready in about 25 minutes. The sweet potatoes will keep you full throughout the morning, and you'll get a good dose of vitamins A and C from the kale. If you want to boost the nutritional profile, add the optional avocado for healthy fat and sprinkle with sesame or hemp seeds.

1 teaspoon avocado oil

2 cups peeled and cubed sweet potatoes

½ cup chopped kale

½ cup diced onion

½ teaspoon sea salt

½ teaspoon freshly ground black pepper

½ avocado, cubed (optional)

1 to 2 teaspoons sesame seeds or
    hemp seeds (optional)

In a large skillet over medium heat, heat the avocado oil. Add the sweet potatoes, kale, onion, salt, and pepper, and sauté for 10 to 15 minutes, or until the sweet potatoes are soft. Remove from the heat.

Gently stir in the avocado and sesame seeds (if using), transfer to 1 large or 2 small plates, and enjoy.

TIP Transform this dish into a breakfast wrap by adding it to a fresh collard green leaf and wrapping like a burrito.

Avocados with Kale and Almond Stuffing

Serves 1 or 2
Prep: 5 minutes
Cook: None

QUICK & EASY

This is a really simple, nutrient-dense breakfast that tastes like it takes much longer to make. The kale and almond stuffing gets its spicy flavor from the jalapeño and a tang from the lemon juice and apple cider vinegar, both of which can help you kick-start your day. The almonds provide a crunchy texture, and the avocado that cradles the stuffing provides a serving of healthy fats to keep you satisfied.

½ cup almonds

½ cup chopped lacinato kale

1 garlic clove

½ jalapeño

2 tablespoons nutritional yeast

1 tablespoon avocado oil

1 tablespoon apple cider vinegar

1 tablespoon freshly squeezed lemon juice

¼ teaspoon sea salt

1 avocado, halved and pitted

In a food processor, pulse the almonds, kale, garlic, jalapeño, nutritional yeast, avocado oil, apple cider vinegar, lemon juice, and sea salt until everything is well combined, the almonds are in small pieces, and it has a chunky texture, taking care not to overprocess.

Add half of the stuffing mixture to the center of each avocado half, and enjoy.

TIP If you have extra time, you can enjoy this as a warm breakfast by baking the avocado in the oven: Just add the stuffed avocado to a baking pan lined with parchment paper and bake at 425°F for 5 to 10 minutes, or until the avocado is soft.

Mixed Berry–Chia Seed Pudding

WEEK 2

Serves 1
Prep: 5 minutes, plus 1 hour to chill
Cook: None

`QUICK & EASY` `NUT-FREE`

This is one of my favorite easy breakfast recipes to make. Make it the night before to let it set in the refrigerator overnight, but you can also make it the same day because it only needs about 1 hour to firm up. Depending on what type of fruit you use (see the tip), you may want to adjust the amount of sweetener.

1 cup coconut milk (boxed)

½ cup mixed berries (raspberries, blackberries, blueberries), plus more (optional) for topping

2 tablespoons chia seeds

1 to 2 tablespoons unrefined whole cane sugar, such as Sucanat

In a mason jar, combine the coconut milk, berries, chia seeds, and sugar, adjusting the sugar to your preference.

Seal the jar tightly, and shake vigorously until well mixed.

Refrigerate for about 1 hour, or until the pudding thickens to your preference.

Stir, top with the extra mixed berries (if using), and enjoy.

TIP This is a versatile recipe. Substitute the mixed berries with your favorite alkaline fruit, like strawberries, mango, bananas, or kiwi.

Pineapple and Coconut Oatmeal Bowl

WEEK 2

Serves 2
Prep: 5 minutes
Cook: 5 minutes

QUICK & EASY   NUT-FREE

Making homemade oatmeal is easier than you think, and much better than prepackaged, store-bought varieties that are usually made by adding hot water. The foundation of this easy breakfast is oatmeal made with full-fat coconut milk, which makes it extra thick and creamy. Canned coconut milk will give the oatmeal the extra-creamy texture that makes this recipe stand out, but feel free to substitute with boxed almond or coconut milk if you prefer.

FOR THE OATMEAL

1 cup quick rolled oats

1 (13.5-ounce) can full-fat coconut milk

2 tablespoons unrefined whole cane sugar, such as Sucanat

FOR ASSEMBLING

½ cup cubed pineapple

¼ cup unsweetened coconut flakes

1 tablespoon chia seeds

1 tablespoon pumpkin seeds, chopped

TO MAKE THE OATMEAL

In a small saucepan over medium-low heat, cook the oats, coconut milk, and sugar for 3 to 5 minutes, or until the oats are soft; adjust the sugar to your preference.

TO ASSEMBLE

Transfer the oatmeal to 2 serving bowls, top with the cubed pineapple, coconut flakes, and chia and pumpkin seeds, and serve.

TIP For a delicious variety to this recipe, substitute the toppings listed above with blueberry Chia Seed Fruit Jam (page 146). Just stir or swirl it into your oatmeal for an extra-special treat!

Oatmeal Porridge with Mango-Chia Fruit Jam

WEEK 2
Serves 2
Prep: 5 minutes
Cook: 5 minutes

`QUICK & EASY` `NUT-FREE`

This homemade oatmeal is easier to make than you think and healthier than prepackaged, store-bought varieties. A couple of spoonfuls of mango Chia Seed Fruit Jam (one of the variations of the Chia Seed Fruit Jam on page 146) makes a colorful topping.

1 (14-ounce) can full-fat coconut milk

1 cup quick rolled oats

2 tablespoons unrefined whole cane sugar, such as Sucanat

1 to 2 tablespoons mango Chia Seed Fruit Jam (page 146)

In a small saucepan over medium-low heat, cook the coconut milk, oats, and sugar, stirring occasionally, for 3 to 5 minutes, or until the oats are soft.

Transfer the oatmeal to 2 serving bowls, top with the mango Chia Seed Fruit Jam, and serve.

TIP Canned coconut will give the oatmeal an extra-creamy texture, but substitute with boxed almond or coconut milk, if you like.

Vanilla Bean and Cinnamon Granola

WEEK 1

Makes 3 cups
Prep: 5 minutes
Cook: 30 minutes

NUT-FREE

Store-bought granola can be expensive, so once you see how easy it is to make granola at home, you'll never go back to purchased granola. After 5 minutes of prep and about 30 minutes in the oven, this granola leaves your kitchen full of the tantalizing, warm aromas of vanilla and cinnamon. It's perfect to enjoy with coconut or almond milk as a quick breakfast or alone as an afternoon snack.

3 cups quick rolled oats

½ cup brown rice syrup

6 tablespoons coconut oil

¼ cup unrefined whole cane sugar, such as Sucanat

2 teaspoons vanilla bean powder

2 teaspoons ground cinnamon

¼ teaspoon sea salt

Preheat the oven to 250°F. Line a baking pan with parchment paper.

In a large bowl, use your hands to mix together the oats, brown rice syrup, coconut oil, sugar, vanilla bean powder, cinnamon, and salt until well combined.

Squeeze the mixture together into a ball, and transfer to the prepared baking pan.

Press the mixture evenly on the baking pan, taking care not to break it up into small pieces. This will allow it to bake in large cluster pieces that you can break apart after baking, if you prefer.

Bake for about 30 minutes, or until crispy, taking care not to overbake.

Cool completely before serving. The granola will harden and get even crispier as it cools. Store in an airtight container.

TIP Customize your granola by adding some sliced almonds, pumpkin seeds, or unsweetened shredded coconut flakes!

Sesame and Hemp Seed Breakfast Cookies

WEEKS 3 & 4

Makes 15 small cookies
Prep: 10 minutes, plus 20 minutes to chill
Cook: None

`QUICK & EASY`

Who says cookies are a bad idea for breakfast? These no-bake breakfast cookies made with sesame and hemp seeds are a great source of plant-based calcium and healthy, balanced omega fatty acids.

⅔ cup cashew butter

½ cup quick rolled oats

¼ cup hemp seeds

¼ cup sesame seeds

3 tablespoons brown rice syrup

3 tablespoons coconut oil, melted

1 teaspoon vanilla bean powder

1 teaspoon ground cinnamon

Line a baking sheet with parchment paper.

In a medium bowl, stir together the cashew butter, oats, hemp seeds, sesame seeds, brown rice syrup, coconut oil, vanilla bean powder, and cinnamon until well combined.

Refrigerate the bowl for 5 to 10 minutes to allow the mixture firm up.

Scoop a tablespoonful of dough at a time and flatten into a disk with your hands. Smooth the outer edges with your fingertips, and place on the prepared baking sheet. Repeat with the remaining dough.

Refrigerate the cookies for about 20 minutes, or until they firm up, and serve. Store leftovers in an airtight container in the refrigerator; they will soften and lose their shape at room temperature.

TIP Another fun way to make this recipe is to take the mixture (a tablespoon at a time) and roll it into the shape of a ball, and instead of a breakfast cookie, you'll have a healthy energy ball to start your day!

Fresh Fruit with Vanilla-Cashew Cream

WEEK 3

Serves 4
Prep: 25 minutes
Cook: None

QUICK & EASY

This divine breakfast of fresh alkaline fruit topped with a pure vanilla-y, cinammony cashew cream is a pretty sweet way to start the morning. Any alkaline fruit will work well—blueberries, strawberries, raspberries, blackberries, mango, pineapple, or cantaloupe—so use whatever you have on hand or is in season.

Room-temperature water, for soaking

1 cup raw cashews

1 (13.5-ounce) can coconut milk

2 tablespoons brown rice syrup

2 tablespoons unrefined whole cane sugar, such as Sucanat

2 teaspoons vanilla bean powder

1 teaspoon freshly squeezed lemon juice

¼ teaspoon ground cinnamon

¼ teaspoon sea salt

4 cups alkaline fruit, such as raspberries, blackberries, blueberries, strawberries, mango, pineapple, or cantaloupe

In a medium bowl with enough room-temperature water to cover them, soak the cashews for 15 to 20 minutes.

Drain and rinse the cashews.

In a high-speed blender, blend to combine the soaked cashews, coconut milk, brown rice syrup, sugar, vanilla bean powder, lemon juice, cinnamon, and salt until creamy and smooth. Add more sugar, if you like.

Add 1 cup of fruit to each of 4 serving bowls, drizzle each bowl of fruit with ½ cup of cream, and serve.

TIP Soaking the cashews softens them, making blending easier. Store any remaining cashew cream in an airtight container in the refrigerator. Add unsweetened shredded coconut flakes over the fruit and cream to make an ambrosia-style dessert.

Pumpkin Seed–Protein Breakfast Balls

WEEKS 1 & 3
Makes 18 to 20 balls
Prep: 5 minutes, plus 20 minutes to chill
Cook: None

QUICK & EASY

These easy no-bake breakfast balls are made with a high-protein ingredient: pumpkin seed protein powder. Pumpkin seed protein powder is cold-pressed and has a complete amino acid profile and a balanced ratio of 3, 6, and 9 fatty acids. These balls can be made in about 5 minutes and only need 15 to 20 minutes to firm up in the refrigerator.

1½ cups quick rolled oats

3 tablespoons 100% organic pumpkin seed protein powder

½ cup almond butter

½ cup raw pumpkin seeds

3 tablespoons brown rice syrup

1 tablespoon coconut oil

1 teaspoon ground cinnamon

1 teaspoon vanilla bean powder

2 to 4 tablespoons coconut milk

Line a baking sheet with parchment paper.

In a food processor, process the oats, protein powder, almond butter, pumpkin seeds, brown rice syrup, coconut oil, cinnamon, vanilla bean powder, and coconut milk until well combined, taking care to not overprocess.

Scoop a tablespoonful into your hands and roll into a ball. Place on the prepared baking sheet, and repeat with the remaining mixture.

Refrigerate for 15 to 20 minutes, or until firm, and serve. Store in the refrigerator; the balls will get soft and lose their shape at room temperature.

***

TIP If you can't find pumpkin seed protein powder, you can omit it.

No-Bake Granola Bars

WEEKS 2 & 3
Makes 6 bars or 12 squares
Prep: 5 minutes, plus 20 minutes to chill
Cook: None

QUICK & EASY

Breakfast on the go couldn't get any easier than these no-bake granola bars that take less than 5 minutes to prepare. Store-bought granola bars typically contain refined sweeteners like high-fructose corn syrup and preservatives. The main ingredient in this healthier version is oats, which are a good source of fiber, with ¼ cup providing 17 percent of your daily value.

1 cup quick rolled oats

½ cup almond butter

2 tablespoons brown rice syrup

1 tablespoon coconut oil

¼ teaspoon sea salt

¼ teaspoon ground cinnamon

¼ teaspoon vanilla bean powder

Line a 9-by-5-inch loaf dish with parchment paper.

In a food processor, process the oats, almond butter, brown rice syrup, coconut oil, salt, cinnamon, and vanilla bean powder until well combined.

Transfer the mixture to the prepared loaf dish, and press down firmly and evenly with your hand and fingertips.

Refrigerate for 15 to 20 minutes, or until the mixture firms up.

Cut into 6 bars or 12 squares, and serve. Store in the refrigerator; the bars will get soft and lose their shape at room temperature.

TIP You can customize these by adding chopped almonds or pumpkin seeds to the mixture after processing.

Blueberry and Chia Seed Cobbler

WEEK 4

Serves 2 to 4
Prep: 5 minutes
Cook: 45 minutes

Traditional blueberry cobbler is made with white flour, refined sugar, and butter, but you won't find any of that in this healthier version. Chia seeds give this comfort food extra fiber and omega-3 fatty acids. You could use this same recipe and substitute the blueberries with mixed berries or even peaches. The recipe calls for a 9-inch oval baking dish, but you could also make individual servings in four (4-ounce) ramekin bowls.

FOR THE BLUEBERRIES

2 cups blueberries

2 tablespoons unrefined whole cane sugar, such as Sucanat

1 tablespoon chia seeds

FOR THE TOPPING

½ cup almond flour

½ cup oat flour

4 tablespoons coconut milk (boxed)

2 tablespoons coconut oil (melted/liquid)

2 tablespoons unrefined whole cane sugar, such as Sucanat

1½ teaspoons baking powder

1 teaspoon vanilla bean powder

¼ teaspoon sea salt

Preheat the oven to 350°F.

TO PREPARE THE BLUEBERRIES

In a medium bowl, stir together the blueberries, sugar, and chia seeds. Transfer the mixture to a 9-inch oval ovenproof baking dish or four (4-ounce) ramekin bowls.

TO PREPARE THE TOPPING

In a medium bowl, stir together the almond flour, oat flour, coconut milk, coconut oil, sugar, baking powder, vanilla bean powder, and salt until well combined.

TO ASSEMBLE

Drop the topping, a tablespoonful at a time, over the blueberry mixture. You can leave the topping as "dollops" or spread it evenly over the top of the blueberry mixture for a full crust.

Bake for 45 minutes, or until the topping is slightly golden and cooked through.

Serve warm.

TIP Make your blueberry cobbler extra special by adding a dollop of Whipped Coconut Cream Topping (page 148).

Frozen Banana–Protein Breakfast Bowl

WEEKS 1 & 3
Serves 1
Prep: 5 minutes, plus overnight to freeze
Cook: None

QUICK & EASY   NUT-FREE

This recipe might seem too simple, but sometimes it's the uncomplicated recipes that pack the most nutrients. With just two ingredients, this quick breakfast bowl packs serious amounts of plant-based protein, as well as a complete amino acid profile and a balanced ratio of healthy 3, 6, and 9 fatty acids. Hemp seeds, chia seeds, or unsweetened shredded coconut flakes add to the nutrition profile.

2 bananas

4 tablespoons pumpkin seed protein powder

Unsweetened shredded coconut flakes, hemp seeds, or chia seeds, for topping (optional)

Peel and slice two bananas, put in a freezer-safe container, and freeze overnight.

In a food processor, process the frozen bananas until they become smooth and creamy with a soft-serve ice cream consistency.

Add the pumpkin protein powder, and process just long enough to mix it in completely.

Transfer to a serving dish, top with the coconut flakes, hemp seeds, or chia seeds (if using), and enjoy.

TIP Always keep frozen sliced bananas in your freezer so you can make this recipe at a moment's notice.

Avocado–Sweet Potato "Toast"

WEEKS 2 & 4

Makes 4 pieces
Prep: 10 minutes
Cook: 10 minutes

`QUICK & EASY` `NUT-FREE`

Now you can enjoy the ever-so-popular "avocado toast" without having to actually eat toast. Instead of using bread, toast a thick slice of sweet potato and top it with a guacamole-inspired topping. This makes a delicious—and nutritious—breakfast.

1 unpeeled sweet potato, cut into
    4 (½-inch-thick) lengthwise slices

2 avocados

½ to 1 jalapeño

2 garlic cloves

1 tablespoon chopped onion

1 tablespoon fresh cilantro leaves

¼ to ½ teaspoon sea salt

Sliced red onion, sliced radish, or dulse flakes,
    for topping (optional)

Place a sweet potato slice in each toaster slot, and toast through about 4 cycles, or until cooked through. They should be tender enough to pierce with a fork. Carefully remove with tongs, and repeat with the remaining slices.

While the sweet potato is toasting, in a food processor, process the avocados, jalapeño, garlic, onion, cilantro, and salt until creamy and smooth. Adjust the salt level as desired.

Spread the avocado topping on top of the sweet potato "toast"; top with the red onion, radish, or dulse flakes (if using); and serve.

TIP For variety, try replacing the avocado topping here with Zucchini and Kale Pesto (page 127).

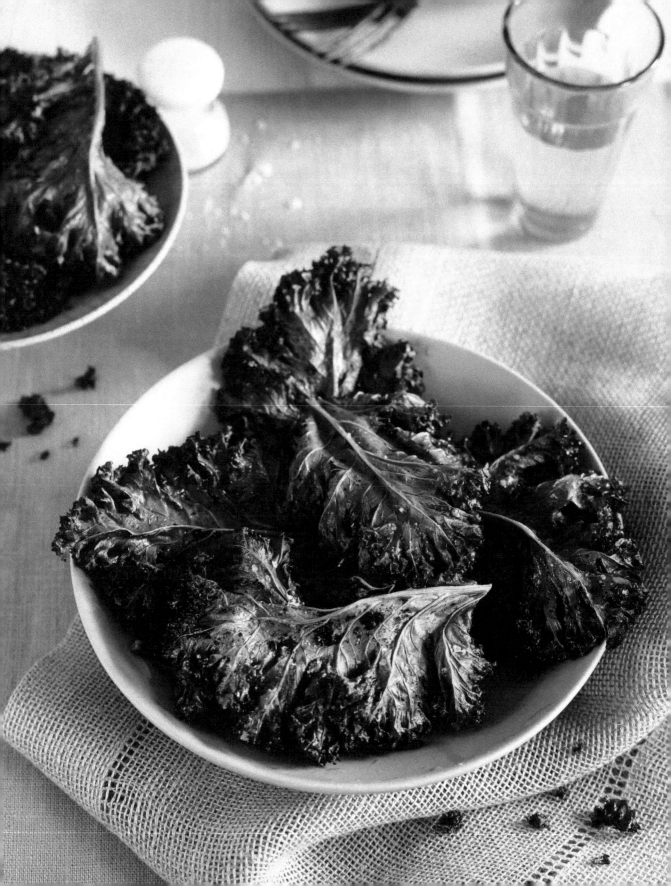

CHAPTER FIVE

DIY Snacks

Tarragon Crackers

WEEKS 1 & 4

Makes 60 small crackers
Prep: 10 minutes
Cook: 15 minutes

QUICK & EASY

These rustic bite-size crackers are perfect when you're craving a savory snack. They're ready in 25 minutes, and the best thing about them is you can substitute the tarragon with your favorite alkaline herb.

3 tablespoons water

1 tablespoon ground flaxseed

2 cups almond flour

1 tablespoon fresh chopped tarragon

1 tablespoon avocado oil

½ teaspoon sea salt

½ teaspoon freshly ground black pepper

¼ teaspoon garlic powder

Preheat the oven to 350°F. Line a baking sheet with parchment paper.

To prepare a flax egg, in a large bowl, whisk together the water and flaxseed.

Add the almond flour, tarragon, avocado oil, salt, pepper, and garlic powder, and stir until well combined.

Transfer the mixture to the prepared baking sheet. Using your hands, form the dough into a ball, then place another piece of parchment paper on the top of the ball.

Using a rolling pin over the parchment paper, roll out the dough to about ¼-inch thickness.

Use a knife or pizza cutter to cut the dough into 60 (1½-inch-by-1½-inch) squares.

Bake for 12 to 14 minutes, or until the crackers are slightly golden on top. Flip them over and bake for another minute or 2.

Cool and serve.

TIP Substitute the tarragon with your favorite alkaline herb like oregano, scallions, dill, or thyme.

Parsley and Tahini Hummus

WEEKS 1, 2 & 3

Makes 1 cup
Prep: 10 minutes
Cook: None

`QUICK & EASY` `NUT-FREE`

High in antioxidants and an anti-inflammatory, parsley ups the flavor and health benefits of this yummy hummus. Dip fresh veggies and Tarragon Crackers (page 68) into it, dress salads with it, and even use it as a spread in wraps.

¼ cup water

2 tablespoons avocado oil

2 teaspoons freshly squeezed lemon juice

3 tablespoons tahini

1 cup chopped fresh parsley sprigs, plus more (optional) for garnish

½ zucchini, peeled

3 garlic cloves, crushed

½ teaspoon sea salt

In a high-speed blender, blend to combine the water, avocado oil, lemon juice, tahini, parsley, zucchini, garlic, and salt until creamy.

Garnish with the extra parsley (if using), and serve.

TIP Tahini is ground-up sesame seeds, and you can either purchase it or make your own, which is really easy. Using a food processor, process 1 cup sesame seeds until they become creamy, and store in an airtight glass jar in the refrigerator. Yields ½ cup tahini.

Paprika-Garlic Almonds

WEEKS 1, 2, 3 & 4
Makes 1 cup
Prep: 5 minutes
Cook: 5 minutes

QUICK & EASY

When the craving for a savory snack hits, these seasoned almonds hit the spot. This stove top method doesn't require waiting around for the oven to heat up. Make sure you get raw almonds and not already roasted or seasoned ones.

1 teaspoon avocado oil

1 cup raw almonds

1 teaspoon ground paprika

½ teaspoon garlic powder

½ to ¾ teaspoon sea salt

In a large skillet over medium heat, heat the avocado oil. Add the almonds, and toss gently until all the almonds are covered with the oil.

Add the paprika, garlic powder, and salt, tossing gently after each addition to make sure it is evenly distributed and all the almonds are covered. Adjust seasonings as desired. Continue cooking and gently tossing for about 5 minutes.

Remove from the heat and allow to cool before serving.

TIP After you remove them from the stove top, toss the almonds with 1 to 2 tablespoons of nutritional yeast for a dairy-free "cheesy" flavor.

Baked Avocado Fries

WEEK 4
Makes 16 fries
Prep: 10 minutes
Cook: 15 minutes

`QUICK & EASY`

Avocado fries are a big hit right now, but they are usually made with flour and eggs and sometimes are even fried. This healthier version is completely oil-free and made with a seasoned almond flour coating and dipped in almond milk instead of eggs. You only need a few simple ingredients to make them, and they're ready in less than 30 minutes. The insides will be soft with the creamy texture of the avocado, and the outsides will have a golden-brown crust.

½ cup almond flour

2 tablespoons nutritional yeast

¼ to ½ teaspoon garlic powder

¼ to ½ teaspoon ground paprika,
    plus more for sprinkling

¼ to ½ teaspoon sea salt

2 avocados, slightly underripe

½ cup almond milk

Preheat the oven to 420°F. Line a baking sheet with parchment paper.

In a small bowl, stir together the almond flour, nutritional yeast, garlic powder, paprika, and salt until well combined.

Halve and pit the avocados, and quarter each half from pole to pole. Peel off the skin.

Add the almond milk to another small bowl.

Dip an avocado slice into first the milk and then the coating mixture, gently tossing it to make sure it is completely covered, and place on the prepared baking sheet. Repeat with the remaining avocado slices.

Bake for 15 to 17 minutes, taking care not to overcook or burn them.

Remove from the oven, sprinkle with additional paprika, and serve immediately.

TIP These pair well with Parsley and Tahini Hummus (page 69), Avocado-Jalapeño Spread (page 117), or Roasted Garlic and Miso Dressing (page 93).

Oregano and Garlic Breadsticks

WEEKS 1, 2 & 3
Makes 12 pieces
Prep: 5 minutes
Cook: 20 minutes

`QUICK & EASY`

These breadsticks are slightly crispy with golden-brown edges and are coated in a savory oregano-garlic topping that will have your kitchen smelling like an Italian pizzeria! They go great with pasta dishes like Zucchini and Kale Pesto Spaghetti Squash (page 127) or Creamy Artichoke and Basil Red Lentil Penne Pasta (page 125), or enjoy them with the Roasted Red Pepper and Artichoke Spread (page 121).

FOR THE BREADSTICKS

3 tablespoons water

1 tablespoon ground flaxseed

2 cups almond flour

1 tablespoon avocado oil

1 tablespoon chopped fresh oregano

½ teaspoon sea salt

½ teaspoon freshly ground black pepper

FOR THE TOPPING

4 garlic cloves, crushed

1 tablespoon chopped fresh oregano

⅛ teaspoon sea salt

⅛ teaspoon freshly ground black pepper

1 tablespoon avocado oil

Preheat the oven to 350°F. Line a baking sheet with parchment paper.

TO PREPARE THE BREADSTICKS

To prepare a flax egg, in a small bowl, whisk together the water and flaxseed until well blended.

In a medium bowl, stir together the flax egg, almond flour, avocado oil, oregano, salt, and pepper until well combined.

Transfer the mixture to the prepared baking sheet, and gather the mixture together to form a ball. Take another sheet of parchment paper, lay it on top of the ball, and using a rolling pin over the paper, roll the dough into a 5-by-8-inch rectangle shape.

TO PREPARE THE TOPPING

In a small bowl, stir together the garlic, oregano, salt, pepper, and avocado oil until well combined. Pour the topping mixture over the dough, and use the back of a spoon to spread it evenly.

Bake for 18 to 20 minutes, or until the edges are golden brown.

Remove from the oven, slice into 12 pieces, and serve.

TIP You can also use the breadstick recipe to make a healthy pizza crust (page 120).

Roasted Okra Bites

Serves 2
Prep: 5 minutes
Cook: 20 minutes

QUICK & EASY   NUT-FREE

There's no need for unhealthy chips or crackers when you're craving a salty snack. All you need are these tasty okra bites that are ready in a pinch, and even better, are super healthy roasted in avocado oil, not the unhealthy oils typically used.

12 okra pods, cut into ¼-inch-thick slices

1 teaspoon avocado oil

½ teaspoon sea salt

¼ teaspoon freshly ground black pepper

Preheat the oven to 450°F. Line a baking sheet with parchment paper.

In a medium bowl, toss the okra and avocado oil to coat. Season with salt and pepper, and toss again.

Place the seasoned okra on the prepared baking sheet in a single layer, and roast for 15 to 20 minutes, flipping halfway through and taking care not to overbake.

These are best served hot from the oven.

TIP Sprinkle these over a salad for a healthy crouton-type topping.

Cheesy Broccoli Bites

WEEKS 1, 3 & 4
Makes 3 cups
Prep: 5 minutes
Cook: 20 minutes

QUICK & EASY

Not only are these bites a tasty snack, they also have loads of nutritional benefits. A half cup of broccoli has 10 percent of your daily value of fiber, 24 percent of your vitamin A, and 84 percent of your vitamin C. Pairing them with nutritional yeast gives you a "cheesy" snack that is dairy-free and ready in just over 20 minutes. Cayenne pepper gives it a little spice, but you can reduce or omit it if you prefer.

½ cup almond flour

½ cup nutritional yeast

½ teaspoon garlic powder

½ teaspoon sea salt

¼ to ½ teaspoon ground cayenne pepper (optional)

3 cups bite-size broccoli florets

2 tablespoons avocado oil

Preheat the oven to 400°F. Line a baking sheet with parchment paper.

In a small bowl, stir together the almond flour, nutritional yeast, garlic powder, salt, and cayenne pepper (if using).

In a medium bowl, toss the broccoli with the avocado oil to coat.

Sprinkle half the seasoning mixture over the broccoli, gently toss until all pieces are coated, and bake for 10 minutes.

Remove from the oven, and transfer the broccoli pieces back to the medium bowl. Sprinkle with the remaining half of the seasoning mix, and toss to coat.

Return to the oven for an additional 5 to 10 minutes, and serve.

TIP Add these bite-size pieces of broccoli to a salad as a healthy replacement for croutons.

Chipotle-Jicama Fries with Scallion Dip

WEEK 2
Serves 2
Prep: 10 minutes
Cook: 40 minutes

Jicama is a root vegetable that can be eaten raw or cooked. In this recipe, we are making a healthy version of fries by oven-baking the jicama and paring it with a creamy scallion dip. You can make the dip while the fries are baking in the oven to save some time. These are best served right out of the oven, but don't worry because you will very likely not have any leftover!

FOR THE JICAMA FRIES

½ jicama, peeled and cut into
    32 (1/4-inch-thick) sticks

1 tablespoon avocado oil

¼ to ½ teaspoon chipotle powder

¼ teaspoon garlic powder

¼ to ½ teaspoon sea salt

¼ teaspoon freshly ground black pepper

FOR THE SCALLION DIP

1½ cups raw cashews

½ cup coconut milk (boxed)

¾ cup roughly chopped scallions

¼ cup vegetable broth

1 tablespoon apple cider vinegar

1 tablespoon freshly squeezed lemon juice

1 garlic clove

½ teaspoon sea salt

Preheat the oven to 400°F. Line a baking sheet with parchment paper.

TO PREPARE THE JICAMA FRIES

In a medium bowl, toss the jicama sticks with the avocado oil to coat.

Add the chipotle powder, garlic powder, salt, and pepper, and toss again to coat. Adjust the seasonings, if necessary.

Transfer the jicama sticks to the prepared baking sheet and spread in a single layer.

Bake for 20 minutes, flip them over, and bake for an additional 15 to 20 minutes.

TO PREPARE THE SCALLION DIP

Meanwhile in a high-speed blender, blend together the cashews coconut milk, scallions, broth, vinegar, lemon juice, garlic, and salt until creamy and smooth. Adjust the seasonings, if necessary, and serve.

TIP The Scallion Dip can also double as a salad dressing: Just add a little extra coconut milk or vegetable broth to give it a thinner consistency.

Cheesy Baked Kale Chips

WEEKS 1, 2, 3 & 4
Serves 1 or 2
Prep: 5 minutes
Cook: 10 minutes

QUICK & EASY   NUT-FREE

Kale chips burst onto the health food scene and have been embraced as a healthy replacement for store-bought chips. This recipe kicks regular kale chips up a notch with nutritional yeast's cheesy taste, giving you deeper satisfaction whenever you crave a salty snack. There are different varieties of kale, but curly kale is best for chips.

4 or 5 stalks curly kale, stemmed and torn
   (2 cups, packed)
1 tablespoon avocado oil
1 tablespoon nutritional yeast
¼ teaspoon sea salt

Preheat the oven to 350°F. Line a baking sheet with parchment paper.

In a medium bowl, toss the kale with the avocado oil to coat.

Sprinkle the nutritional yeast and salt over the kale, and toss to coat.

Transfer the kale to the prepared baking sheet, and bake for 5 to 6 minutes. Turn them over and bake for an additional 5 to 6 minutes, or until they are crispy, taking care not to burn them.

Cool and serve.

TIP These are also great to crumble over a salad as a topping.

Lemon and Garlic Cashew Cream–Stuffed Mushrooms

WEEKS 1, 2 & 4
Makes 12 mushrooms
Prep: 5 minutes
Cook: 5 minutes

QUICK & EASY

These cute stuffed mushrooms are an easy snack plus a tasty and super quick choice for hors d'oeuvres. Lightly sautéed baby portobello (cremini) mushrooms are filled with a tangy lemon cashew cream that's a breeze to pull together. For a second hors d'oeuvres choice, fill the baby bellas with Zucchini and Kale Pesto (page 127).

FOR THE MUSHROOMS

12 cremini mushrooms, stemmed

1½ teaspoons avocado oil

Pinch sea salt

Pinch freshly ground black pepper

FOR THE STUFFING

1 cup raw cashews

2 garlic cloves

¼ cup freshly squeezed lemon juice

1 teaspoon apple cider vinegar

¼ teaspoon sea salt

TO PREPARE THE MUSHROOMS

Rinse and dry the mushroom caps.

In a medium skillet over medium heat, heat the avocado oil. Add the mushroom caps, sprinkle with salt and pepper, and sauté for 2 to 4 minutes, or until they soften. Discard any liquid that may accumulate.

TO PREPARE THE STUFFING

In a high-speed blender, blend to combine the cashews, garlic, lemon juice, vinegar, and salt until a thick paste forms.

Spoon the stuffing mixture evenly among the 12 mushroom caps and serve.

TIP The stuffing here has all the hallmarks of a delicious pasta sauce. Add a bit of water while the blender is still going to create a luscious pasta sauce, and top with a dash fresh lemon zest.

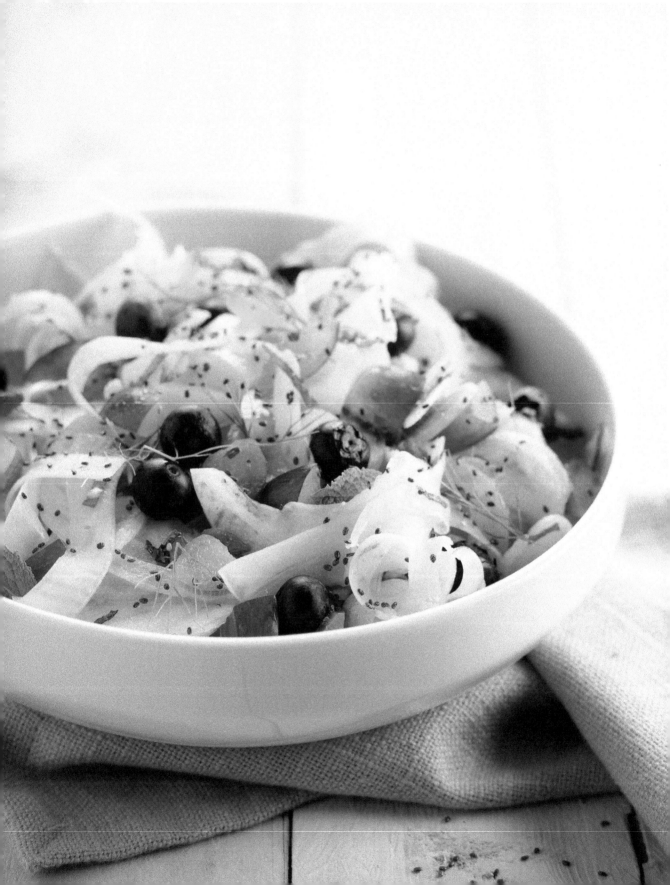

CHAPTER SIX

Meal-Size Salads

Warm Asparagus Salad with Lemon-Asparagus Dressing

WEEK 2

Serves 1 or 2
Prep: 10 minutes
Cook: 5 minutes

QUICK & EASY

A warm salad can be a nice change of pace from traditional salads, and this one is really easy to make with only two steps: a quick sauté of the asparagus followed by blending the dressing. Asparagus, a high-alkaline vegetable, is the star of the show, but paired with the tangy Lemon-Asparagus Dressing, this truly is a high-alkaline meal you can enjoy with only nine healthy ingredients.

FOR THE SALAD

1 teaspoon avocado oil

24 asparagus stalks, diced

½ cup diced onion

3 garlic cloves, crushed

½ teaspoon sea salt

¼ teaspoon freshly ground black pepper

FOR THE DRESSING

½ cup raw cashews

½ cup water

2 tablespoons freshly squeezed lemon juice

¼ teaspoon sea salt

⅛ teaspoon freshly ground black pepper

FOR ASSEMBLING

2 cups mixed salad greens

TO PREPARE THE ASPARAGUS MIXTURE

In a large skillet over medium heat, heat the avocado oil. Add the asparagus, onion, garlic, salt, and pepper, and sauté for 5 to 7 minutes, or until the onion is soft.

TO PREPARE THE DRESSING

In a high-speed blender, blend together half the asparagus mixture with the cashews, water, lemon juice, salt, and pepper until creamy and smooth.

TO ASSEMBLE THE SALAD

Plate the mixed salad greens on 1 large or 2 small plates. Top with the remaining asparagus mixture, drizzle with the dressing, and enjoy.

TIP Give your salad a nutritional boost by garnishing with hemp seeds or sesame seeds.

Warm Sweet Potato Salad with Jalapeño-Cilantro Dressing

WEEK 3

Serves 1 or 2
Prep: 10 minutes
Cook: 25 minutes

With more fiber, potassium, and vitamin A than white potatoes, sweet potatoes are a perfect addition to a healthy salad. Mixed salad greens work well here, but feel free to use your favorite greens, like kale, romaine, red leaf lettuce, or even arugula. The Jalapeño-Cilantro Dressing ties it all together with a bit of heat.

FOR THE SWEET POTATOES

3 medium sweet potatoes, peeled and cubed

2 tablespoons avocado oil

2 garlic cloves, crushed

1 teaspoon ground paprika

½ teaspoon sea salt

FOR THE JALAPEÑO-CILANTRO DRESSING

1 cup water

1 cup raw cashews

¼ cup fresh cilantro leaves

½ to 1 jalapeño

2 tablespoons freshly squeezed lime juice

½ teaspoon sea salt

FOR ASSEMBLING

2 cups mixed salad greens

Preheat the oven to 350°F. Line a baking sheet with parchment paper.

TO PREPARE THE SWEET POTATOES

In a medium bowl, toss together the sweet potatoes, avocado oil, garlic, paprika, and salt.

Spread the sweet potato cubes evenly on the prepared baking pan, and bake for 25 minutes, or until soft.

TO PREPARE THE JALAPEÑO-CILANTRO DRESSING

Meanwhile, in a high-speed blender, blend together the water, cashews, cilantro, jalapeño, lime juice, and salt until smooth.

TO ASSEMBLE

Plate the mixed salad greens on 1 large or 2 small plates. Top with the warm sweet potatoes, drizzle with the dressing, and enjoy.

TIP Make a double batch of the Jalapeño-Cilantro Dressing to use for another salad or even as a dip for the Baked Avocado Fries on page 71.

Pineapple Salad with Lime Vinaigrette

WEEK 3
Serves 1 or 2
Prep: 10 minutes
Cook: None

QUICK & EASY   NUT-FREE

The tart and tangy lime vinaigrette in this salad goes perfectly with the sweet pineapple, the star of the show. Purple cabbage and limes are both excellent sources of vitamin C and are rich in antioxidants. Mixed salad greens or a spring mix offer a variety of different greens that you might not normally purchase separately, like green and red leaf lettuce, red and green chard, arugula, green oak leaf, mizuna, tatsoi, and lolla rosa.

FOR THE LIME VINAIGRETTE

¼ cup avocado oil

¼ cup water

2 tablespoons freshly squeezed lime juice

½ cup chopped scallions

½ cup chopped fresh cilantro

2 garlic cloves

½ teaspoon sea salt

FOR ASSEMBLING

2 to 3 cups mixed salad greens

½ cup cubed pineapple

1 cup chopped purple cabbage

Dulse flakes, for garnish (optional)

TO PREPARE THE VINAIGRETTE

In a blender, blend together the avocado oil, water, lime juice, onion, cilantro, garlic, and salt until well combined. Adjust the seasonings, if necessary.

TO ASSEMBLE THE SALAD

Plate the mixed salad greens on 1 large or 2 small plates. Top with the pineapple, purple cabbage, and dulse flakes (if using); drizzle with the dressing; and serve.

TIP If you don't have fresh pineapple, canned pineapple will work, too. Just make sure it doesn't have any added sugar.

Peach Salsa Salad with Sweet Tahini Dressing

WEEK 2

Serves 1 or 2
Prep: 10 minutes
Cook: None

`QUICK & EASY` `NUT-FREE`

Using fresh peaches in this light and colorful salad (instead of tomatoes as the base, as with traditional salsa) transforms a well-loved sauce into an excellent topping for a healthy salad. The peaches add a little sweetness, balancing out the familiar salsa flavors of cilantro, onions, and jalapeño.

FOR THE DRESSING

4 tablespoons tahini

3 to 4 tablespoons brown rice syrup

¼ cup water

1 teaspoon freshly squeezed lemon juice

Pinch sea salt

FOR THE SALSA

1 peach, pitted and cubed

¼ cup diced red bell pepper

1 tablespoon chopped fresh cilantro

1 tablespoon diced red onion

½ jalapeño, diced

FOR ASSEMBLING

2 to 3 cups mixed salad greens

TO PREPARE THE DRESSING

In a small bowl, whisk together the tahini, brown rice syrup, water, lemon juice and salt until well combined. Adjust seasonings, if necessary.

TO PREPARE THE SALSA

In another small bowl, toss together the peach, bell pepper, cilantro, onion, and jalapeño.

TO ASSEMBLE THE SALAD

Plate the mixed salad greens on 1 large or 2 small plates. Top with the salsa, drizzle with the dressing, and enjoy.

TIP You can also enjoy the peach salsa as a regular salsa.

Red Lentil Penne Pasta Salad with Sautéed Vegetables

WEEKS 1 & 4
Serves 2 to 4
Prep: 15 minutes
Cook: 15 minutes

QUICK & EASY   NUT-FREE

Pasta salad is an excellent vehicle for summer's abundance of produce. For pasta, use red lentil penne pasta, made from 100-percent organic red lentils. A protein powerhouse, the pasta has 21 grams of plant-based protein in one 3-ounce serving.

FOR THE PASTA AND DRESSING

2 cups red lentil pasta

¼ cup avocado oil

2 tablespoons apple cider vinegar

1 tablespoon freshly squeezed lemon juice

1 teaspoon dried oregano

2 pinches sea salt

2 pinches freshly ground black pepper

FOR THE VEGGIES

1 tablespoon avocado oil

6 asparagus stalks, diced

1 cup diced orange bell pepper

⅓ cup diced red onion

½ zucchini, sliced

½ summer squash, sliced

2 garlic cloves, crushed

TO PREPARE THE PASTA AND DRESSING

Cook the pasta according to package directions.

While the pasta cooks, in a small bowl, whisk together the avocado oil, vinegar, lemon juice, oregano, salt, and pepper until well combined. Adjust the seasonings, if necessary.

TO PREPARE THE VEGGIES

In a skillet over medium-high heat, heat the avocado oil. Add the asparagus, bell pepper, onion, zucchini, squash, and garlic, and sauté for 2 to 3 minutes, or just until soft.

TO ASSEMBLE

In a large bowl, toss the cooked pasta, veggies, and dressing until well combined. Transfer to 2 large or 4 small plates and enjoy.

TIP If you can't find red lentil pasta, this would also be good to enjoy with just the sautéed veggies and dressing by itself, over a bed of mixed salad greens or spaghetti squash pasta.

Chopped Veggie Salad with Spicy Avocado-Cream Dressing

Serves 2
Prep: 10 minutes
Cook: None

`QUICK & EASY`

Light and colorful, this salad is made with fresh veggies and topped with a spicy avocado-based dressing. Both the dressing and veggies are spicy from the jalapeños, but you can reduce or omit them and still have a vibrant, healthy salad to enjoy. And, you can substitute the bell pepper and onions with your favorite variety.

FOR THE DRESSING

1 avocado, roughly chopped

1 cup fresh cilantro

2 garlic cloves

½ to 1 jalapeño

2 tablespoons water

1 tablespoon freshly squeezed lime juice

1 teaspoon avocado oil

½ teaspoon sea salt

FOR THE VEGGIES

½ orange bell pepper

¼ cup red onion

1 medium carrot

½ cup broccoli florets

½ to 1 jalapeño

FOR ASSEMBLING

2 to 4 cups mixed salad greens

TO PREPARE THE DRESSING

In a blender, blend together the avocado, cilantro, garlic, jalapeño, water, lime juice, avocado oil, and salt until creamy and smooth. Adjust the seasonings if necessary.

TO PREPARE THE VEGGIES

In a food processor, process the bell pepper, onion, carrot, broccoli, and jalapeño until they are chopped into tiny pieces, taking care not to overprocess.

TO ASSEMBLE

In a medium bowl, toss together the salad greens and veggies. Transfer the salad to 2 plates, drizzle with the dressing, and enjoy.

TIP Add extra nutrients by sprinkling some dulse flakes over the top.

Roasted Artichoke Salad with Sesame Seed Vinaigrette

Serves 1 or 2
Prep: 5 minutes
Cook: 30 minutes

NUT-FREE

Artichokes aren't just delicious; they boast many nutritional benefits. One cup of artichoke hearts contains more antioxidants than blueberries, cranberries, and even cooked broccoli! Artichokes are also an excellent source of dietary fiber, having more fiber than prunes and oats. In this salad, roasted artichokes top salad greens and a tangy sesame seed vinaigrette dressing is drizzled over for a top-notch healthy meal.

FOR THE ARTICHOKES

1 (14-ounce) can artichoke hearts, drained

1 tablespoon avocado oil

⅛ teaspoon sea salt

⅛ teaspoon freshly ground black pepper

⅛ teaspoon garlic powder

⅛ teaspoon ground paprika

FOR THE DRESSING

2 tablespoons avocado oil

2 tablespoons apple cider vinegar

1 tablespoon sesame seeds

1 tablespoon brown rice syrup

1 shallot, diced

⅛ teaspoon sea salt

⅛ teaspoon freshly ground black pepper

FOR ASSEMBLING

2 to 4 cups mixed salad greens

Preheat the oven to 425°F. Line a baking sheet with parchment paper.

TO PREPARE THE ARTICHOKES

Cut off the artichoke tips, and then cut each heart in half. Rub avocado oil all over the artichoke pieces.

In a small bowl, mix together the salt, pepper, garlic, and paprika. Place the artichokes on the prepared baking sheet, and sprinkle the seasoning over them, tossing to coat.

Roast the artichoke pieces for 30 minutes, tossing halfway through.

TO PREPARE THE DRESSING

While the artichokes are roasting, in a small bowl, whisk together the avocado oil, vinegar, sesame seeds, brown rice syrup, shallot, salt, and pepper until well blended. Adjust the seasonings, if necessary.

TO ASSEMBLE

In a large bowl, toss the artichokes with the mixed salad greens and drizzle with the dressing. Transfer to 1 large or 2 small plates and enjoy.

TIP The roasted artichokes are great to enjoy by themselves as a snack.

Roasted Beet–Kale Salad with Lemon-Garlic Vinaigrette

WEEK 2

Serves 1 or 2
Prep: 10 minutes
Cook: 20 minutes

`QUICK & EASY` `NUT-FREE`

An antioxidant-rich and anti-inflammatory food, beets are a tasty pairing to the kale in this salad. Massaging kale with your hands is the easiest way to make it softer and milder in flavor, while keeping all the antioxidants that kale can lose during cooking. You'll know it's ready when it transforms right before your eyes, shrinking and becoming slightly wilted.

FOR THE BEETS

4 small beets, peeled and cut into small cubes

1 teaspoon avocado oil

¼ teaspoon dried rosemary

⅛ teaspoon garlic powder

Pinch sea salt

Pinch freshly ground black pepper

FOR THE KALE

2 cups bite-size stemmed curly kale pieces

⅛ teaspoon sea salt

FOR THE DRESSING

2 tablespoons avocado oil

1 tablespoon freshly squeezed lemon juice

1 tablespoon brown rice syrup

1 garlic clove, crushed

Pinch sea salt

Pinch freshly ground black pepper

Preheat the oven to 400°F. Line a baking pan with parchment paper.

TO PREPARE THE BEETS

In a small bowl, toss the beets with the avocado oil to coat. Sprinkle with the rosemary, garlic powder, salt, and pepper, and toss to coat. Transfer the beets to the prepared baking pan and roast for 15 to 20 minutes, or until slightly crispy.

TO PREPARE THE KALE

Meanwhile, in a medium bowl, sprinkle the kale with the salt, and gently massage the kale with your hands, scrunching it until it becomes soft and slightly limp, about 3 minutes. Transfer to a serving dish.

TO PREPARE THE DRESSING

In a small bowl, whisk together the avocado oil, lemon juice, brown rice syrup, garlic, salt, and pepper until well combined.

TO ASSEMBLE

Add the beets to the bowl with the kale, and drizzle with the dressing. Transfer to 1 large or 2 small plates and enjoy.

TIP If you're short on time, just skip the roasting process and add the uncooked seasoned beets to your salad!

Mushroom-Lentil Salad with Lime-Tahini Dressing

WEEKS 1, 3 & 4
Serves 1 or 2
Prep: 5 minutes
Cook: 25 minutes

`QUICK & EASY` `NUT-FREE`

This savory mushroom and lentil combo complements the sautéed shallots and garlic. Use leftover lentils if you have them—they are an excellent source of plant-based protein (1 cup has 36 percent of your daily value) and also boast an impressive amount of fiber (63 percent of your daily value).

FOR THE MUSHROOM-LENTIL MIXTURE

⅓ cup dry lentils

1 tablespoon avocado oil

6 cremini mushrooms, sliced

1 tablespoon chopped shallot

1 garlic clove, crushed

Pinch sea salt

Pinch freshly ground black pepper

FOR THE DRESSING

2 tablespoons tahini

1 tablespoon freshly squeezed lime juice

1 teaspoon avocado oil

3 tablespoons water

Pinch salt

Pinch freshly ground black pepper

FOR ASSEMBLING

2 to 4 cups mixed salad greens

TO PREPARE THE MUSHROOM-LENTIL MIXTURE

Prepare the lentils according to package directions.

In a large skillet over medium-high heat, heat the avocado oil. Add the cooked lentils (you'll need 1 cup), mushrooms, shallot, garlic, salt, and pepper, and sauté for 2 to 4 minutes, or until the mushrooms are soft.

TO PREPARE THE DRESSING

In a small bowl, whisk together the tahini, lime juice, avocado oil, water, salt, and pepper until well combined.

TO ASSEMBLE

Plate the mixed salad greens on 1 large or 2 small plates. Top with the mushroom-lentil mixture, drizzle with the dressing, and enjoy.

TIP Save time by making a double batch of lentils so you can use them for more than one recipe!

Roasted Carrot and Onion Salad with Creamy Cashew-Miso Dressing

WEEKS 1 & 4
Serves 1 or 2
Prep: 5 minutes
Cook: 30 minutes

`QUICK & EASY`

Seasoned and roasted carrots and red onions are layered on top of a bed of spicy arugula greens and paired with a creamy miso dressing. The base for the dressing is cashew butter with an added touch of miso, which is a high-alkaline, unpasteurized fermented food. If you like raw carrots, you can slice or shred them and dice the onions to save time and make this a raw meal.

FOR THE ROASTED VEGETABLES

2 carrots, sliced

½ cup thinly sliced red onion

1 teaspoon avocado oil

Pinch sea salt

Pinch freshly ground black pepper

Pinch garlic powder

FOR THE DRESSING

2 tablespoons cashew butter

2 teaspoons organic white miso

3 tablespoons water

Pinch freshly ground black pepper

FOR ASSEMBLING

2 to 4 cups arugula

Preheat the oven to 425°F. Line a baking pan with parchment paper.

TO PREPARE THE VEGGIES

In a medium bowl, toss the carrots and onion in the avocado oil to coat. Season with salt, pepper, and garlic powder.

Transfer to the prepared baking pan, and roast for 25 to 30 minutes, or until the carrots and onion are soft.

TO PREPARE THE DRESSING

Meanwhile, in a small bowl, whisk together the cashew butter, miso, water, and pepper until well combined. Miso is a high-sodium food so the dressing shouldn't need any sea salt, but try it and add salt, if necessary.

TO ASSEMBLE

Plate the arugula on 1 large or 2 small plates. Top with the roasted veggies, drizzle with the dressing, and enjoy.

TIP If you can't find organic white miso, you can omit it and add sea salt; the dressing will still work well with this salad.

Cashew-Broccoli Salad with Spicy Cashew Dressing

WEEK 1

Serves 1 or 2
Prep: 5 minutes
Cook: 20 minutes

`QUICK & EASY`

Replace traditional peanut sauce with alkaline cashew butter and added red pepper flakes for a bit of heat, which balances beautifully with the creamy dressing. Cashews are an excellent source of copper (¼ cup has 98 percent of your daily value), and broccoli is a great source of fiber (1 cup has 21 percent of your daily value).

FOR THE BROCCOLI

2 cups bite-size broccoli florets

1 teaspoon avocado oil

Pinch sea salt

Pinch freshly ground black pepper

Pinch garlic powder

FOR THE DRESSING

¼ cup cashew butter

1 tablespoon apple cider vinegar

1 tablespoon coconut aminos

1 tablespoon brown rice syrup

1 tablespoon red pepper flakes

¼ teaspoon avocado oil

2 to 3 tablespoons water

FOR ASSEMBLING

2 to 4 cups mixed salad greens

¼ cup raw cashews

3 tablespoons chopped scallions

2 teaspoons sesame seeds

Preheat the oven to 400°F. Line a baking sheet with parchment paper.

TO PREPARE THE BROCCOLI

In a small bowl, toss the broccoli with the avocado oil to coat. Season with the salt, pepper, and garlic powder.

Transfer the broccoli to the prepared baking sheet, and roast for 15 to 20 minutes, or until the broccoli is soft.

TO PREPARE THE DRESSING

Meanwhile, in a small bowl, whisk together the cashew butter, vinegar, aminos, brown rice syrup, red pepper flakes, avocado oil, and water until well combined.

TO ASSEMBLE

Plate the mixed greens one 1 large or 2 small plates, and top with the roasted broccoli, cashews, and scallions. Drizzle with the dressing, garnish with the sesame seeds, and enjoy.

TIP Coconut aminos is a healthy replacement for soy sauce. It doesn't contain soy, has 73 percent less sodium, and contains 17 naturally occurring amino acids. Use it in any recipe that calls for soy sauce.

Watermelon-Basil Salad with Basil Vinaigrette

WEEK 4

Serves 1 or 2
Prep: 10 minutes
Cook: None

`QUICK & EASY` `NUT-FREE`

Watermelon is such a hydrating fruit, and this light and colorful salad is the perfect blend of sweet and tangy. The basil vinaigrette gets its tartness from apple cider vinegar, which perfectly complements the sweetness of the watermelon. This no-cook salad is ideal when you don't want to heat the kitchen or need a quick lunch.

½ cup fresh basil leaves, plus 8 fresh
   basil leaves, chopped

¼ cup avocado oil

¼ cup apple cider vinegar

1 garlic clove

¼ teaspoon sea salt

2 to 4 cups mixed salad greens

2 cups cubed watermelon

In a blender, blend together the basil, avocado oil, vinegar, garlic, and salt until well combined.

Plate the salad greens on 1 large or 2 small plates. Top with the cubed watermelon, sprinkle with the chopped basil, drizzle with the vinaigrette, and enjoy.

TIP This is also great as a light snack, without the salad greens. Just fill a bowl with cubed watermelon and chopped basil, and drizzle with the vinaigrette.

Creamy Green Olive Pasta Salad

WEEK 2

Serves 1 or 2
Prep: 10 minutes
Cook: None

QUICK & EASY

This easy pasta salad brings together 100 percent organic red lentil pasta and a creamy, plant-based dressing. A 3-ounce serving of this dish provides 21 grams of protein, and the green olives are packed with antioxidants and vitamin E.

FOR THE DRESSING

½ cup raw cashews

1 cup coconut milk (boxed)

1 tablespoon apple cider vinegar

2 garlic cloves

⅛ teaspoon dried dill

½ to ¾ teaspoon sea salt

FOR ASSEMBLING

2 cups cooked lentil pasta

2 tablespoons sliced green olives

2 tablespoons chopped scallions

TO PREPARE THE DRESSING

In a blender, blend together the cashews, coconut milk, vinegar, garlic, dill, and salt until well combined. Adjust the salt, if necessary.

TO ASSEMBLE

Transfer the cooked pasta to a medium bowl, add the dressing, green olives, and scallions, and toss until well combined. Plate the salad on 1 large or 2 small plates and enjoy.

TIP This pasta salad can be enjoyed as a warm or cold salad.

Blueberry and Fennel Salad with Roasted Garlic and Miso Dressing

WEEK 4
Serves 1
Prep: 10 minutes
Cook: None

NUT-FREE

This light and summery salad combines high-antioxidant blueberries with aromatic fennel. You'll want to make sure you slice the fennel as thin a possible so the taste isn't overpowering. The dressing is very versatile and great to keep on hand. It has the deep, aromatic flavor of roasted garlic and the distinct taste of miso, both of which are high in nutrients and health benefits. If you preplan and use frozen roasted garlic cloves, you can make this recipe in less than 10 minutes.

FOR THE DRESSING

1 head Roasted Garlic (page 150)

½ cup avocado oil

¼ cup water

2 tablespoons organic white miso

2 tablespoons freshly squeezed lime juice

1 teaspoon ground black pepper

FOR THE SALAD

2 cups mixed salad greens

½ cup blueberries

¼ cup finely sliced fennel

1 tablespoon fresh mint leaves

1 to 2 teaspoons chia seeds, for garnish

TO PREPARE THE DRESSING

In a blender, blend together 8 of the roasted garlic cloves with the avocado oil, water, miso, lime juice, and pepper until well combined and smooth. Adjust seasonings to your preference.

TO PREPARE THE SALAD

Add the mixed salad greens to your serving bowl, and top with the blueberries, fennel, mint, and chia seeds.

Drizzle the salad dressing over the top, or add it to the salad and toss it in so the entire salad is covered with the dressing.

Garnish with chia seeds and enjoy.

TIP The Roasted Garlic and Miso Dressing is so versatile—try it as a pasta sauce over red lentil pasta, a dip for veggies, drizzled over a baked sweet potato, or in a wrap.

Fresh Herb Potato Salad

WEEK 2

Serves 1 or 2
Prep: 10 minutes
Cook: 20 minutes

QUICK & EASY   NUT-FREE

However you prepare them, including in a potato salad, potatoes are considered by most to be one of, if not *the*, most popular comfort foods. This recipe gives traditional potato salad a healthier makeover with a tangy and flavorful herb-based dressing. It has lots of color and crunch from the radishes and the scallions and red onion. Potatoes also happen to be a good source of fiber (1 cup provides 15 percent of your daily value).

2 cups peeled and diced small white potatoes

FOR THE DRESSING

¼ cup fresh parsley

¼ cup chopped scallions

1 celery stalk

¼ cup avocado oil

1 tablespoon freshly squeezed lime juice

2 teaspoons apple cider vinegar

2 garlic cloves

½ to ¾ teaspoon sea salt

FOR ASSEMBLING

1 radish, sliced

2 tablespoons chopped scallions

2 tablespoons diced red onion

TO PREPARE THE POTATOES

In a medium saucepan, cover the potatoes with water about 2 inches over the top of the potatoes. Boil for 18 to 20 minutes, or until the potatoes are soft.

Drain and transfer to a medium bowl.

TO PREPARE THE DRESSING

Meanwhile, in a blender, blend together the parsley, scallions, celery, avocado oil, lime juice, vinegar, garlic, and salt until well combined. Adjust the seasonings, if necessary.

TO ASSEMBLE

Pour the dressing over the potatoes, and gently stir until the dressing is evenly distributed, taking care not to mash the potatoes too much.

Gently stir in the radish, scallions, and red onion; transfer to 1 large or 2 small plates; and enjoy.

TIP You can enjoy this potato salad warm or cold.

Peach Salad with Sweet Citrus Dressing

Serves 1 large or 2 small
Prep: 10 minutes
Cook: 0 minutes

`QUICK & EASY` `NUT-FREE`

This fresh fruit salad is not only bright and colorful, but the blueberries and peaches also provide a healthy dose of antioxidants and fiber. The dressing has a sweet and tangy flavor from fresh squeezed orange and lime juice and doesn't have any added oil. Chopped romaine lettuce is a light and mild-flavored leafy green, but feel free to use your favorite alkaline salad greens.

FOR THE DRESSING

2 tablespoons orange juice (fresh squeezed)

1 tablespoon lime juice (fresh squeezed)

1 tablespoon brown rice syrup

1 pinch sea salt

FOR ASSEMBLING

2–4 cups chopped romaine leaves

1 cup cubed peaches

8 large basil leaves, cut into long, thin strips

TO PREPARE THE DRESSING

In a small bowl, whisk together the orange and lemon juices, brown rice syrup, and salt until well combined. Adjust seasonings to your preference.

TO ASSEMBLE

In a serving dish, add the chopped romaine leaves, sprinkle the peaches over the top, and drizzle with the dressing. Transfer to 1 large or 2 small plates, garnish each serving with some of the basil, and enjoy.

TIP Add some texture and crunch to your salad by sprinkling slivered almonds on top!

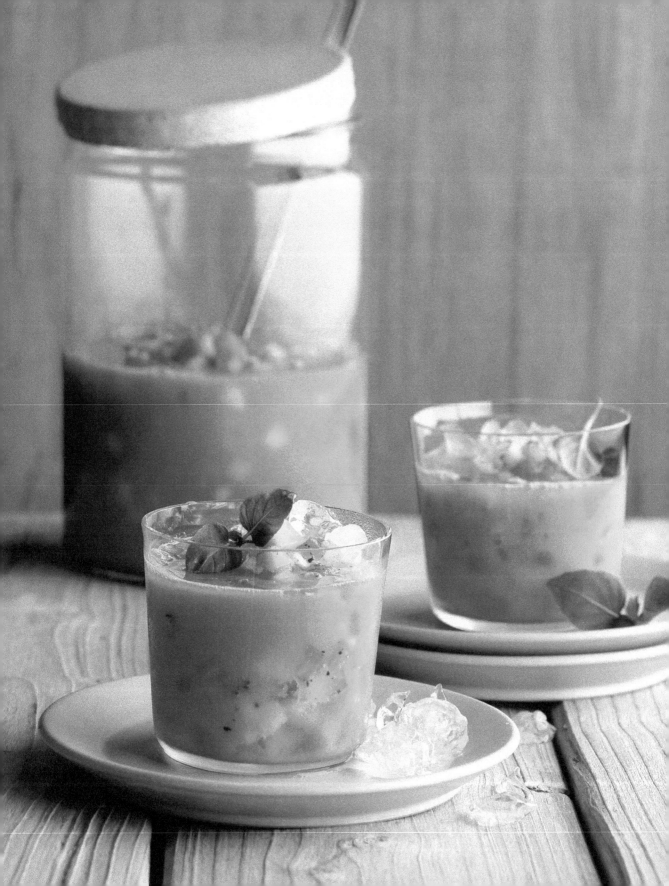

CHAPTER SEVEN

Soups and Stews

Lemon-Tarragon Soup

Serves 1 or 2
Prep: 10 minutes
Cook: 10 minutes

QUICK & EASY

Cashews and coconut milk replace heavy cream in this healthy version of lemon-tarragon soup, balanced by tart freshly squeezed lemon juice and fragrant tarragon. It's a light, airy soup that you won't want to miss.

1 tablespoon avocado oil

½ cup diced onion

3 garlic cloves, crushed

¼ plus ⅛ teaspoon sea salt

¼ plus ⅛ teaspoon freshly ground black pepper

1 (13.5-ounce) can full-fat coconut milk

1 tablespoon freshly squeezed lemon juice

½ cup raw cashews

1 celery stalk

2 tablespoons chopped fresh tarragon

In a medium skillet over medium-high heat, heat the avocado oil. Add the onion, garlic, salt, and pepper, and sauté for 3 to 5 minutes, or until the onion is soft.

In a high-speed blender, blend together the coconut milk, lemon juice, cashews, celery, and tarragon with the onion mixture until smooth. Adjust seasonings, if necessary.

Pour into 1 large or 2 small bowls and enjoy immediately, or transfer to a medium sauce-pan and warm on low heat for 3 to 5 minutes before serving.

TIP This soup would pair well with the Tarragon Crackers on page 68.

Chilled Cucumber and Lime Soup

Serves 1 or 2
Prep: 5 minutes, plus 20 minutes to chill
Cook: None

QUICK & EASY   NUT-FREE

Chilled soups are perfect for the hot summer months, and this easy soup is made with garden fresh vegetables with no cooking involved. Simply prep the veggies, add them to a blender, and lunch is served! If your produce is coming out of the refrigerator, you may not need to chill the soup after making it, but if not, just place it in the refrigerator to enjoy chilled later or even the next day.

1 cucumber, peeled

½ zucchini, peeled

1 tablespoon freshly squeezed lime juice

1 tablespoon fresh cilantro leaves

1 garlic clove, crushed

¼ teaspoon sea salt

In a blender, blend together the cucumber, zucchini, lime juice, cilantro, garlic, and salt until well combined. Add more salt, if necessary.

Pour into 1 large or 2 small bowls and enjoy immediately, or refrigerate for 15 to 20 minutes to chill before serving.

TIP This recipe could also double as a healthy dip for freshly sliced veggies!

Coconut, Cilantro, and Jalapeño Soup

WEEK 3

Serves 1 or 2
Prep: 5 minutes
Cook: 5 minutes

`QUICK & EASY` `NUT-FREE`

This soup is a nutrient dream. Cilantro is a natural anti-inflammatory and is also excellent for detoxification. And one single jalapeño has an entire day's worth of vitamin C! Add to this healthy combination fresh garlic, onion, and citrusy lime juice, and you have an easy soup that you can feel good about eating.

2 tablespoons avocado oil

½ cup diced onions

3 garlic cloves, crushed

¼ teaspoon sea salt

1 (13.5-ounce) can full-fat coconut milk

1 tablespoon freshly squeezed lime juice

½ to 1 jalapeño

2 tablespoons fresh cilantro leaves

In a medium skillet over medium-high heat, heat the avocado oil. Add the onion, garlic, and salt, and sauté for 3 to 5 minutes, or until the onions are soft.

In a blender, blend together the coconut milk, lime juice, jalapeño, and cilantro with the onion mixture until creamy.

Pour into 1 large or 2 small bowls and enjoy.

TIP A versatile soup, it can be enjoyed immediately out of the blender, chilled, or lightly warmed over low heat.

Spicy Watermelon Gazpacho

Serves 1 or 2
Prep: 5 minutes
Cook: None

QUICK & EASY **NUT-FREE**

At first taste, this soup may have you wondering if you're lunching on a hot and spicy salsa. It has the heat and seasonings of a traditional tomato-based salsa, but it also has a faint sweetness from the cool watermelon. The soup is really hot with a whole jalapeño, so if you don't like food too hot, just use half a jalapeño.

2 cups cubed watermelon

¼ cup diced onion

¼ cup packed cilantro leaves

½ to 1 jalapeño

2 tablespoons freshly squeezed lime juice

In a blender or food processor, pulse to combine the watermelon, onion, cilantro, jalapeño, and lime juice only long enough to break down the ingredients, leaving them very finely diced and taking care to not overprocess.

Pour into 1 large or 2 small bowls and enjoy.

TIP This recipe also doubles as a healthy salsa-type dip, but without tomatoes!

Roasted Carrot and Leek Soup

WEEK 2

Serves 2 to 4
Prep: 10 minutes
Cook: 30 minutes

The carrot, a root vegetable, is an excellent source of antioxidants (1 cup has 113 percent of your daily value of vitamin A) and fiber (1 cup has 14 percent of your daily value). This bright and colorful soup freezes well to enjoy later when you're short on time.

6 carrots

1 cup chopped onion

1 fennel bulb, cubed

2 garlic cloves, crushed

2 tablespoons avocado oil

1 teaspoon sea salt

1 teaspoon freshly ground black pepper

2 cups almond milk, plus more if desired

Preheat the oven to 400°F. Line a baking sheet with parchment paper.

Cut the carrots into thirds, and then cut each third in half. Transfer to a medium bowl.

Add the onion, fennel, garlic, and avocado oil, and toss to coat. Season with the salt and pepper, and toss again.

Transfer the vegetables to the prepared baking sheet, and roast for 30 minutes.

Remove from the oven and allow the vegetables to cool.

In a high-speed blender, blend together the almond milk and roasted vegetables until creamy and smooth. Adjust the seasonings, if necessary, and add additional milk if you prefer a thinner consistency.

Pour into 2 large or 4 small bowls and enjoy.

TIP This soup would work great as a sauce over spaghetti squash or even roasted cauliflower.

Creamy Lentil and Potato Stew

WEEKS 1, 2, 3 & 4

Serves 4
Prep: 10 minutes
Cook: 30 minutes

`QUICK & EASY` `NUT-FREE`

This is a hearty stew that is sure to be a favorite. It's a one-pot meal that is the perfect comfort food. With fresh vegetables and herbs along with protein-rich lentils, it's both healthy and filling. Any lentil variety would work, even a mixed, sprouted lentil blend. Another bonus of this recipe: It's freezer-friendly.

2 tablespoons avocado oil

½ cup diced onion

2 garlic cloves, crushed

1 to 1½ teaspoons sea salt

1 teaspoon freshly ground black pepper

1 cup dry lentils

2 carrots, sliced

1 cup peeled and cubed potato

1 celery stalk, diced

2 fresh oregano sprigs, chopped

2 fresh tarragon sprigs, chopped

5 cups vegetable broth, divided

1 (13.5-ounce) can full-fat coconut milk

In a large soup pot over medium-high heat, heat the avocado oil. Add the onion, garlic, salt, and pepper, and sauté for 3 to 5 minutes, or until the onion is soft.

Add the lentils, carrots, potato, celery, oregano, tarragon, and 2½ cups of vegetable broth, and stir.

Bring to a boil, reduce the heat to medium-low, and cook, stirring frequently and adding additional vegetable broth a half cup at a time to make sure there is enough liquid for the lentils and potatoes to cook, for 20 to 25 minutes, or until the potatoes and lentils are soft.

Remove from the heat, and stir in the coconut milk. Pour into 4 soup bowls and enjoy.

TIP Want a brothy soup? Just omit the coconut milk, and you'll still enjoy the rustic flavors of this healthy stew.

Roasted Garlic and Cauliflower Soup

WEEKS 3 & 4
Serves 1 or 2
Prep: 10 minutes
Cook: 35 minutes

Roasted garlic is always a treat, and paired with cauliflower in this wonderful soup, what you get is a deeply satisfy soup with savory, rustic flavors. Blended, the result is a smooth, thick, and creamy soup, but if you prefer a thinner consistency, just add a little more vegetable broth to thin it out. Cauliflower is anti-inflammatory, high in antioxidants, and a good source of vitamin C (1 cup has 86 percent of your daily value).

4 cups bite-size cauliflower florets

5 garlic cloves

1½ tablespoons avocado oil

¾ teaspoon sea salt

½ teaspoon freshly ground black pepper

1 cup almond milk

1 cup vegetable broth, plus more if desired

Preheat the oven to 450°F. Line a baking sheet with parchment paper.

In a medium bowl, toss the cauliflower and garlic with the avocado oil to coat. Season with the salt and pepper, and toss again.

Transfer to the prepared baking sheet, and roast for 30 minutes. Cool before adding to the blender.

In a high-speed blender, blend together the cooled vegetables, almond milk, and vegetable broth until creamy and smooth. Adjust the salt and pepper, if necessary, and add additional vegetable broth if you prefer a thinner consistency.

Transfer to a medium saucepan, and lightly warm on medium-low heat for 3 to 5 minutes.

Ladle into 1 large or 2 small bowls and enjoy.

TIP Add some extra nutrients by garnishing your soup with some high-alkaline dulse flakes.

Beefless "Beef" Stew

WEEKS 1 & 4
Serves 4
Prep: 10 minutes
Cook: 50 minutes

NUT-FREE

The potatoes, carrots, aromatics, and herbs in this soup meld so well together, you'll forget there's typically beef in this stew. Hearty and flavorful, this one-pot comfort food is perfect for a fall or winter dinner.

1 tablespoon avocado oil

1 cup onion, diced

2 garlic cloves, crushed

1 teaspoon sea salt

1 teaspoon freshly ground black pepper

3 cups vegetable broth, plus more if desired

2 cups water, plus more if desired

3 cups sliced carrot

1 large potato, cubed

2 celery stalks, diced

1 teaspoon dried oregano

1 dried bay leaf

In a medium soup pot over medium heat, heat the avocado oil. Add the onion, garlic, salt, and pepper, and sauté for 2 to 3 minutes, or until the onion is soft.

Add the vegetable broth, water, carrot, potato, celery, oregano, and bay leaf, and stir. Bring to a boil, reduce the heat to medium-low, and cook for 30 to 45 minutes, or until the potatoes and carrots are soft.

Adjust the seasonings, if necessary, and add additional water or vegetable broth, if a soupier consistency is preferred, in half-cup increments.

Ladle into 4 soup bowls and enjoy.

TIP Make Oregano and Garlic Breadsticks (page 72) to go with this dish.

Creamy Mushroom Soup

Serves 2 to 4
Prep: 5 minutes
Cook: 20 minutes

QUICK & EASY   **NUT-FREE**

This savory, earthy soup is a must try if you love mushrooms. Shiitake and baby portobello (cremini) mushrooms are used here, but you can substitute them with your favorite mushroom varieties. Full-fat coconut milk gives it that close-your-eyes-and-savor-it creaminess that pushes the soup into the comfort food realm—perfect for those cold evenings when you need a warm soup to heat up your insides.

1 tablespoon avocado oil

1 cup sliced shiitake mushrooms

1 cup sliced cremini mushrooms

1 cup diced onion

1 garlic clove, crushed

¾ teaspoon sea salt

½ teaspoon freshly ground black pepper

1 cup vegetable broth

1 (13.5-ounce) can full-fat coconut milk

½ teaspoon dried thyme

1 tablespoon coconut aminos

In a large soup pot over medium-high heat, heat the avocado oil. Add the mushrooms, onion, garlic, salt, and pepper, and sauté for 2 to 3 minutes, or until the onion is soft.

Add the vegetable broth, coconut milk, thyme, and coconut aminos. Reduce the heat to medium-low, and simmer for about 15 minutes, stirring occasionally.

Adjust seasonings, if necessary, ladle into 2 large or 4 small bowls, and enjoy.

TIP The Tarragon Crackers on page 68 would go perfectly with this soup! See the tip on page 90 for more information on coconut aminos.

Chilled Berry and Mint Soup

Serves 1 or 2
Prep: 5 minutes, plus 20 minutes to chill
Cook: None

QUICK & EASY **NUT-FREE**

There's no better way to cool down when it's hot outside than with this chilled, sweet mixed berry soup. It's light and showcases summer's berry bounty: raspberries, blackberries, and blueberries. The fresh mint brightens the soup and keeps the sweetness in check. This soup isn't just for lunch or dinner either—try it for a quick breakfast, too! If you prefer a thinner consistency, just add a little extra water.

FOR THE SWEETENER

¼ cup unrefined whole cane sugar,
   such as Sucanat

¼ cup water, plus more if desired

FOR THE SOUP

1 cup mixed berries (raspberries, blackberries,
   blueberries)

½ cup water

1 teaspoon freshly squeezed lemon juice

8 fresh mint leaves

TO PREPARE THE SWEETENER

In a small saucepan over medium-low, heat the sugar and water, stirring continuously for 1 to 2 minutes, until the sugar is dissolved. Cool.

TO PREPARE THE SOUP

In a blender, blend together the cooled sugar water with the berries, water, lemon juice, and mint leaves until well combined.

Transfer the mixture to the refrigerator and allow to chill completely, about 20 minutes.

Ladle into 1 large or 2 small bowls and enjoy.

TIP Save time and use frozen berries so you can enjoy the soup right away without having to wait for it to chill!

Broccoli and Potato Soup

WEEK 4

Serves 2 to 4
Prep: 10 minutes
Cook: 25 minutes

NUT-FREE

Even if you aren't a big fan of broccoli, you have to try this thick and creamy soup. The broccoli flavor is very subtle and mild, and the soup's depth comes from the potatoes and coconut milk. Broccoli is an excellent source of vitamins K and C and is high in fiber (1 cup cooked broccoli has 21 percent of your daily value).

1 tablespoon avocado oil

½ cup diced onion

2 garlic cloves, crushed

3 cups vegetable broth

1 (13.5-ounce) can full-fat coconut milk

2 cups peeled and cubed potatoes

3 cups bite-size broccoli florets

1 teaspoon sea salt

1½ teaspoons freshly ground black pepper

In a large skillet over medium-high heat, heat the avocado oil. Add the onion and garlic, and sauté for 2 to 3 minutes, or until the onions are soft.

Add the vegetable broth, coconut milk, potatoes, broccoli, salt, and pepper, and continue to cook for 18 to 20 minutes, or until the potatoes are soft. Remove from the heat and cool.

In a blender, blend the cooled soup until smooth.

Adjust the seasonings, if necessary. Pour into 2 large or 4 small bowls and enjoy.

TIP Sprinkle 1 or 2 teaspoons of nutritional yeast on top to give it a "cheesy" flavor!

Spicy Chilled Red Pepper Soup

WEEK 3

Serves 2 to 4
Prep: 5 minutes, plus 30 minutes to chill
Cook: 10 minutes

NUT-FREE

This spicy soup has a flavorful base of red bell peppers and sautéed onions and garlic. It also has extra diced pieces of fresh red and yellow bell peppers added in for texture. It's a great "make-ahead" soup because the flavors actually intensify after chilling overnight in the refrigerator. Start with half a jalapeño, or even omit it completely, if you prefer less heat.

1 teaspoon avocado oil

¼ cup diced onions

2 garlic cloves, crushed

2 cups diced red bell peppers

2 cups vegetable broth

½ to 1 jalapeño, seeded and diced

1 teaspoon sea salt

½ cup small-diced red bell peppers

½ cup small-diced yellow bell peppers

To a skillet over medium-high heat, add the avocado oil, onions, garlic, and red bell peppers, and sauté for 2 to 3 minutes, or until the onions are soft; allow to cool.

In a blender, blend together the sautéed mixture, vegetable broth, jalapeño, and salt until everything is well combined and completely liquid; adjust seasonings to your preference.

Transfer the soup to a medium bowl, and stir in the diced red and yellow bell peppers.

Cover and refrigerate for 20 to 30 minutes to cool or chill overnight.

Ladle into 2 large or 4 small bowls and enjoy.

TIP For an enticing visual presentation, add some crushed ice cubes to the top of your soup before serving!

French Onion and Kale Soup

Serves 2 to 4
Prep: 10 minutes
Cook: 20 minutes

QUICK & EASY

This nondairy version of the classic French Onion Soup has all the signature deep, savory flavors and none of the typical dairy ingredients. It has a vegetable broth base, and the onions are lightly caramelized, rendering them soft and melt-in-your-mouth flavorful. The kale gives the soup a nutritional boost as an excellent source of vitamins A, C, and K.

1 tablespoon avocado oil

2 cups thinly sliced yellow onions (3 medium)

1 teaspoon unrefined whole cane sugar, such as Sucanat

1 cup vegetable broth

2 cups water

2 tablespoons coconut aminos

2 garlic cloves, crushed

½ teaspoon dried thyme

½ teaspoon sea salt

3 kale stalks, stemmed and cut into ribbons (about 2 cups)

In a medium soup pot over medium-high heat, heat the avocado oil. Add the onions and sauté for 3 to 5 minutes, or until the onions begin to get soft.

Add the sugar and continue to sauté, stirring continuously, for 8 to 10 minutes, or until the onions are slightly caramelized.

Add the vegetable broth, water, coconut aminos, garlic, thyme, and salt. Reduce the heat to medium-low, and simmer for 5 to 7 minutes. Adjust seasonings, if necessary.

Add the kale and leave over the heat just long enough for the kale to wilt.

Remove from the heat, ladle into 2 large or 4 small bowls, and serve.

TIP Yellow onions work best for this soup, but for variety, feel free use a combination of 1 cup yellow onions and 1 cup red onions.

Wild Rice and Mushroom-Miso Soup

WEEK 1

Serves 1 to 2
Prep: 10 minutes
Cook: 55 minutes

NUT-FREE

A quick glance at the ingredient list for this recipe might make you wonder where the flavor comes from in this earthy broth-like soup. Not only does the broth get its flavor from the tender mushrooms and leeks, but once you add the miso, it just bursts with flavor. This is a good recipe to make if you have leftover wild rice, since it only needs 1 cup. Once the wild rice is prepared, the soup is ready in only about 10 minutes from start to finish.

⅓ cup wild rice

1 cup sliced cremini mushrooms

½ cup sliced leeks, white part only

3 cups water

2 tablespoons organic white miso

¼ to ½ teaspoon freshly ground black pepper

Sliced scallions, for garnish

Prepare the wild rice according to the package directions.

In a medium soup pot over high heat, bring the sliced mushrooms, leeks, and water to a boil. Boil for 8 to 10 minutes, or until the mushrooms are soft.

Add the cooked wild rice, miso, and black pepper. Using the back side of a spoon, mash the miso on the side of the pot to break it down, and then stir it in.

Remove from the heat. Ladle into 1 large or 2 small bowls, garnish with the chopped scallions, and enjoy.

TIP Since miso is a high-sodium food, this soup doesn't have added sea salt, but if you prefer, adjust the seasonings to your preference.

Ginger and Pear Soup

Serves 1 to 2
Prep: 10 minutes
Cook: 15 minutes

QUICK & EASY   NUT-FREE

This is a delicate and light soup with the mild sweetness of pears and a faint hint of ginger. Because of the many health benefits ginger provides, it's a good soup to make to help with any type of digestive issues, including nausea. This soup is also a good source of fiber from the pears, with one medium pear having 6 grams per serving. The ginger isn't overpowering in this recipe, but if you like the strong, hot flavor of ginger, feel free to add more.

2 teaspoons avocado oil

½ cup diced onions

2 garlic cloves, crushed

1 cup vegetable broth

2 cups water

¼ cup coconut milk (boxed)

2 peeled and cubed pears

1-inch piece fresh ginger root, minced

¼ teaspoon sea salt

Sliced radishes, for garnish (optional)

Chopped scallions, for garnish (optional)

In a large skillet over medium-high heat, heat the avocado oil. Add the onion and garlic, and sauté for 2 to 3 minutes, or until the onions are soft.

Add the vegetable broth, water, coconut milk, pears, ginger, and salt, and cook on medium-high heat for 8 to 10 minutes, or until the pears are soft. Remove from the heat and cool.

Transfer the soup to a blender, and blend until well combined. Adjust seasonings, if necessary.

Pour immediately into 1 large or 2 small bowls, garnish with the radishes and scallions (if using), and enjoy, or return the soup to the stove top to lightly warm on low heat before serving.

TIP You can enjoy this soup chilled, at room temperature, or lightly warmed on the stove top.

Artichoke and Asparagus Soup

Yields: 4 cups
Prep: 5 minutes
Cook: 20 minutes

QUICK & EASY

Creamy asparagus soup is delicious just by itself, but the artichoke gives it a slightly tart flavor. Asparagus is an anti-inflammatory and antioxidant food that also provides an amazing 101 percent DV of Vitamin K in 1 cup. Artichokes are also an excellent antioxidant food and a good source of dietary fiber. This easy soup is great to make on a cold day, and it's freezer-friendly, too!

½ cup diced onion

1 tablespoon avocado oil

2 garlic cloves, crushed

1 cup cubed potatoes

8 stalks asparagus, cut into bite-size pieces

2 cups vegetable broth

½ to ¾ teaspoon sea salt

½ teaspoon ground black pepper

2 cups almond milk

1 can artichoke hearts, stemmed and halved

In a medium skillet, sauté the onion, avocado oil, and garlic over medium-high heat for 2 to 3 minutes, or until the onion is soft.

Transfer the sautéed mixture to a medium-size saucepan and add the potatoes, asparagus, vegetable broth, salt, and pepper; simmer over medium-high heat for 18 to 20 minutes, or until the potatoes are soft. Add extra vegetable broth, if needed, to keep the liquid level between ½ to 1 inch over the contents in the saucepan. Remove from the heat and allow to cool.

In a blender, blend the cooled soup mixture, almond milk, and artichokes until everything is well combined and the soup is smooth. Adjust seasonings to your preference and add extra almond milk or vegetable broth to thin it out, if you prefer.

Return the soup to the saucepan and lightly warm on low heat before serving.

TIP Substitute the almond milk with coconut milk—2 cups boxed coconut milk or one (13.5-ounce) can of full-fat coconut milk—to make this a nut-free recipe.

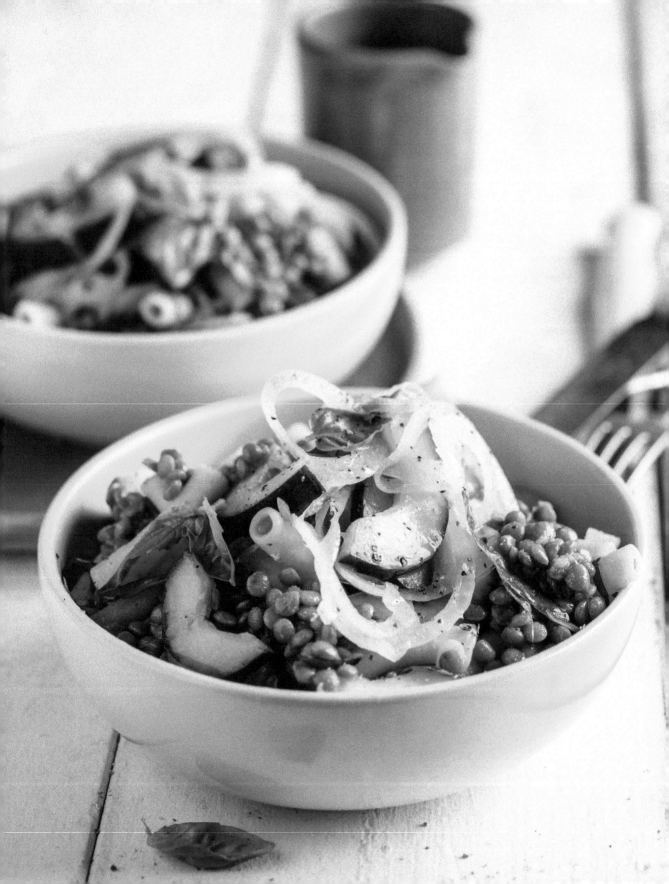

CHAPTER EIGHT

Mains

Spicy Eggplant Stir-Fry

WEEKS 1 & 4

Serves 2 to 4
Prep: 10 minutes
Cook: 5 minutes

`QUICK & EASY` `NUT-FREE`

This one-skillet meal isn't just quick and easy, it also takes advantage of two of summer's fresh veggies—eggplant and bell peppers. Not only is it great to enjoy by itself, it's also delicious in a fresh collard green leaf wrap or over a bed of salad greens. It's a little spicy, so you may want to start with ¼ teaspoon of black pepper, adding more as necessary.

3 tablespoons avocado oil

3 cups cubed eggplant (about three-quarters of an eggplant)

2 tablespoons coconut aminos

2 garlic cloves, crushed

½ teaspoon sea salt

½ teaspoon freshly ground black pepper

½ orange bell pepper, diced

½ yellow bell pepper, diced

½ red bell pepper, diced

Chopped scallions and/or sesame seeds, for garnish (optional)

In a large skillet over medium-high heat, heat the avocado oil. Add the eggplant, coconut aminos, garlic, salt, and pepper, and sauté for 3 to 5 minutes, or until the eggplant is soft.

Reduce the heat to low, add the bell peppers, and toss just long enough for everything to be coated.

Remove from the heat, transfer to 2 large or 4 small plates, and serve garnished with scallions and/or sesame seeds (if using).

TIP Try adding the stir-fry to red lentil penne pasta or even spaghetti squash for variety.

Nori Veggie Rolls with Avocado-Jalapeño Spread

WEEKS 1 & 4
Makes 2 large rolls
Prep: 10 minutes
Cook: None

`QUICK & EASY` `NUT-FREE`

High-alkaline nori sheets are most commonly used in sushi, but they can also be used to make healthy rolls like these. Rolls are a great way to incorporate veggies into a meal. The nori sheets and a fresh collard green leaf are filled with colorful veggies and a fresh avocado spread with a little spice from a jalapeño.

FOR THE AVOCADO-JALAPEÑO SPREAD

1 avocado, pitted and halved

¼ cup fresh cilantro leaves

2 tablespoons freshly squeezed lemon juice

½ to 1 jalapeño

¼ teaspoon sea salt

FOR THE ROLLS

2 collard green leaves

2 nori sheets

½ red bell pepper, sliced

½ orange bell pepper, sliced

½ yellow bell pepper, sliced

½ cup chopped purple cabbage

2 tablespoons chopped fresh cilantro leaves

TO PREPARE THE AVOCADO-JALAPEÑO SPREAD

In a blender, blend together the avocado, cilantro, lemon juice, jalapeño, and salt until smooth.

TO PREPARE THE ROLLS

Lay 1 collard green leaf flat, and place 1 nori sheet on top of it.

Spread half the avocado-jalapeño mixture down the center.

Take half of the bell peppers, cabbage, and cilantro, and arrange in the center of the nori sheet on the avocado-jalapeño spread. Roll like a burrito. Repeat with the remaining collard green leaf, nori, bell pepper, cabbage, and cilantro.

Enjoy each roll whole or halved.

TIP You can also make a "deconstructed" vegetable roll by turning it into a salad: Just break the nori sheet into small pieces, stem and chop the collard greens, and add both to a salad bowl. Then toss with the veggie filling and use the jalapeño spread as a dressing!

Lentil and Sweet Potato Taco Wraps

WEEKS 1 & 4
Makes 2 wraps
Prep: 10 minutes
Cook: 30 minutes

`NUT-FREE`

These hearty taco wraps are made with a spicy lentil filling topped with seasoned baked sweet potato cubes nestled in a fresh collard green wrap. This dish is perfect to try with the Nondairy Sour Cream recipe (page 144). It takes about 5 minutes to make, and you won't regret it after your first taste!

FOR THE SWEET POTATO

1 sweet potato, peeled and cut into
    bite-size cubes

2 teaspoons avocado oil

1 garlic clove, crushed

⅛ teaspoon ground paprika

⅛ teaspoon sea salt

FOR THE LENTILS

¾ cup dry lentils, cooked according to
    package directions

1 cup fresh cilantro leaves

½ to 1 jalapeño

1 tablespoon avocado oil

1 tablespoon freshly squeezed lemon juice

2 garlic cloves, crushed

1 teaspoon sea salt

½ teaspoon freshly ground black pepper

FOR ASSEMBLING

2 collard green leaves

Nondairy Sour Cream (page 144), for garnish
    (optional)

Preheat the oven to 350°F.

TO PREPARE THE SWEET POTATO

In a small bowl, toss the sweet potato with the avocado oil to coat. Add the garlic, paprika, and salt, and toss to coat again. Bake for 25 to 30 minutes, or until soft.

TO PREPARE THE LENTILS

In a food processor, pulse the cooked lentils, cilantro, jalapeño, avocado oil, lemon juice, garlic, salt, and pepper until well combined, taking care to not overprocess.

TO ASSEMBLE

Spread half the lentil mixture onto a collard green leaf, top it with half the sweet potatoes, and drizzle with Nondairy Sour Cream (if using). Repeat with the remaining lentils, collard green leaf, sweet potatoes, and Nondairy Sour Cream, and enjoy.

TIP Want to save some time? Substitute the baked sweet potato cubes with cubed or sliced avocado.

Cheesy Scallop Potato and Onion Bake

WEEKS 1, 2, 3 & 4

Serves 4
Prep: 10 minutes
Cook: 45 minutes

These oven-baked potato slices are covered with the creamy nondairy cheese sauce. Traditional scallop potato recipes tend to be a bit on the heavier side, so with a few healthy substitutions, this classic comfort food is transformed into an alkaline dish you can enjoy.

8 small new potatoes, sliced thin

1½ onions, diced small

1 tablespoon avocado oil

1 teaspoon sea salt

1 teaspoon freshly ground black pepper

1 tablespoon chopped fresh tarragon

1 recipe Cashew Cheese Sauce (page 145)

Preheat the oven to 375°F

In a large bowl, mix the potatoes and onions with the avocado oil to coat. Add the salt, pepper, and tarragon, and toss again.

In an 8-by-8-inch baking dish, layer the potatoes in 3 rows. Overlap and stand them up as necessary to fit in the dish. Sprinkle the diced onions between the potato slices and rows.

Bake for about 45 minutes, or until the potatoes are soft.

Remove from the oven, and pour the cheese sauce over the potatoes. Transfer to 4 plates and enjoy immediately, or return the baking dish to the oven to warm the sauce for 5 minutes before serving.

TIP Change this recipe up by using sliced sweet potatoes instead! Just bake at 350°F for 30 minutes, or until they become soft.

Fresh Veggie Pizza with Tahini-Beet Spread

WEEKS 2 & 3
Makes 4 small pieces
Prep: 10 minutes
Cook: 15 minutes

`QUICK & EASY`

This easy flat bread–style pizza is so versatile, you'll want to add it to your weekly recipe rotation. You can top it with any of your favorite fresh, sautéed, or roasted veggies; the possibilities are truly endless. Instead of the traditional tomato sauce, this tangy, creamy tahini-beet spread is full of vibrant color and flavor. You can also use the Broccoli-Basil Pesto (page 123) for a little variety.

FOR THE CRUST

1¼ cup almond flour

3 tablespoons coconut oil

½ teaspoon sea salt

½ teaspoon garlic powder

FOR THE TAHINI-BEET SPREAD

2 beets, peeled and cubed

1 tablespoon tahini

1 tablespoon avocado oil

1 tablespoon freshly squeezed lemon juice

2 garlic cloves

⅛ teaspoon sea salt

Pinch freshly ground black pepper

FOR ASSEMBLING

Mushrooms, red onions, dandelion greens, asparagus, jalapeños, artichokes, arugula, broccoli, basil, dulse flakes (optional toppings)

Preheat the oven to 375°F. Line a baking sheet with parchment paper.

TO PREPARE THE CRUST

In a small bowl, stir together the almond flour, coconut oil, salt, and garlic powder until well combined.

Transfer to the prepared baking pan, and squeeze the mixture together until it forms a ball shape. Lay another sheet of parchment paper on top of the ball, and use a rolling pin to roll the dough out over the parchment paper into a 7-by-7-inch square.

Bake for about 14 minutes, until the edges turn golden brown.

TO PREPARE THE TAHINI-BEET SPREAD

Meanwhile, in a food processor, process the beets, tahini, avocado oil, lemon juice, garlic, salt, and pepper until thick and creamy. Adjust the seasonings, if necessary.

TO ASSEMBLE

When the crust is ready, spread the tahini-beet spread evenly over it, top the pizza with your favorite alkaline veggies, cut into 4 slices, and enjoy.

TIP The Tahini-Beet Spread would also work great as a salad dressing—just add 1 to 2 tablespoons of water to thin it out.

Sweet Potato Slices with Roasted Red Pepper and Artichoke Spread

WEEKS 1 & 3
Makes 8 pieces
Prep: 5 minutes
Cook: 45 minutes

NUT-FREE

In this recipe, thick slices of sweet potato are baked and then topped with a tangy, savory roasted red bell pepper and artichoke spread. The bell pepper and sweet potatoes can be roasted in the oven at the same time, and the spread takes less than 5 minutes to make to complete the meal.

2 unpeeled sweet potatoes, cut into 4 (¼-inch-thick) lengthwise slices

1 red bell pepper, quartered

6 teaspoons avocado oil, divided

½ teaspoon salt, plus 1 pinch

¼ teaspoon freshly ground black pepper, plus 1 pinch

1 (14-ounce) can artichoke hearts

2 garlic cloves

Preheat the oven to 350°F. Line a baking sheet with parchment paper.

Transfer the sweet potato and bell pepper to the prepared baking sheet, and drizzle with 2 teaspoons of avocado oil, the pinch salt, and the pinch pepper.

Bake for 30 minutes. Flip them over and return to the oven for an additional 15 minutes.

In a food processor, pulse the roasted red bell pepper, the remaining 4 teaspoons of avocado oil, the remaining ½ teaspoon of salt, the remaining ¼ teaspoon of black pepper, the artichoke hearts, and the garlic until well combined but still chunky. Adjust seasonings, if necessary.

Top the sweet potato slices with the spread and enjoy.

TIP The Roasted Red Pepper and Artichoke Spread would be great to add to a salad or even use as a dip for fresh veggies.

Roasted Cauliflower Wraps with Mango-Habanero Sauce

WEEKS 1 & 3
Makes 2 wraps
Prep: 5 minutes
Cook: 35 minutes

`NUT-FREE`

This recipe shows how versatile cauliflower is. Here, it's coated in a gluten-free breading, roasted, wrapped with mixed salad greens, and topped with a sweet and hot mango-habanero sauce. Habanero peppers are very hot, so if you have never tried one before, you may want to start with only a half of the pepper.

FOR THE CAULIFLOWER AND BREADING

2 cups bite-size cauliflower florets
1 tablespoon avocado oil
¼ cup almond flour
¼ cup nutritional yeast
½ teaspoon garlic powder
¼ teaspoon sea salt
¼ teaspoon freshly ground black pepper

FOR THE SAUCE

1 cup cubed mango
1 habanero pepper
2 garlic cloves
2 tablespoons apple cider vinegar
⅛ teaspoon sea salt

FOR ASSEMBLING

½ to 1 cup mixed salad greens
2 fresh collard green leaves

Preheat the oven to 350°F. Line a baking sheet with parchment paper.

TO PREPARE THE CAULIFLOWER AND BREADING

In a medium bowl, toss the cauliflower with the avocado oil to coat.

In a small bowl, stir together the almond flour, nutritional yeast, garlic powder, salt, and pepper until well combined.

Add the breading mixture to the cauliflower, and toss until all pieces are covered. Transfer to the prepared baking sheet.

Roast the cauliflower for 30 to 35 minutes, or until soft.

TO PREPARE THE SAUCE

Meanwhile, in a blender, blend together the mango, habanero, garlic, vinegar, and salt until well combined. (Take extra precautions when handling the habanero pepper: Use rubber gloves or wash your hands thoroughly after handling.)

TO ASSEMBLE

Place half of the mixed salad greens in the center of a collard green leaf, top it with half of the cauliflower, drizzle the sauce on top, and wrap like a burrito. Repeat to make the second wrap, and enjoy.

TIP Turn this wrap into a salad—just omit the collard green leaf, add the roasted cauliflower to a bed of alkaline greens, and top with the mango-habanero sauce!

Stuffed Sweet Potato with Broccoli-Basil Pesto

WEEKS 2 & 4

Makes 2 potatoes
Prep: 10 minutes
Cook: 1 hour, 15 minutes

A baked sweet potato stuffed with fresh, raw, dairy-free pesto is a filling and satisfying meal. The pesto is so flavorful you could eat it on its own, especially as a healthy alternative to the typical butter and cheese toppings for stuffed potatoes. In a pinch, white potatoes, which are also alkaline, can sub for sweet potatoes if you don't have any on hand.

2 large sweet potatoes

2½ cups broccoli

2½ cups almonds

½ cup fresh basil leaves

¼ cup onion

2 garlic cloves

2 tablespoon avocado oil

¼ cup nutritional yeast

½ teaspoon sea salt

Preheat the oven to 350°F.

Pierce the sweet potatoes all over with a fork. Place the sweet potatoes on a baking sheet, and bake for 1 hour and 15 minutes, or until they are soft.

Meanwhile, prepare the pesto. In a food processor, pulse the broccoli, almonds, basil, onion, garlic, avocado oil, nutritional yeast, and salt until the broccoli and almonds are ground into tiny pieces. Adjust the seasonings, if necessary.

When the potatoes are ready, cut them in half lengthwise, and gently scoop out the insides of the potato, taking care not to tear the potato skin; add the baked potato filling to a medium bowl, and add the pesto mixture; gently stir together.

Divide the mixture in half, add each half back into the two empty potato skins, and serve.

TIP The Broccoli-Basil Pesto is a great alternative for a topping in the pizza recipe on page 120, or as a spread on a wrap or even as a dip for fresh veggies!

Lentil and Cucumber Pasta Bowl

WEEKS 1 & 3
Serves 1 or 2
Prep: 5 minutes
Cook: None

QUICK & EASY   NUT-FREE

This is a filling and satisfying meal loaded with plant-based protein from the lentils and green lentil pasta. They are tossed together and then topped with fresh, cool cucumbers, thinly sliced onions, and a tangy vinaigrette-style dressing with fresh basil leaves. Save time by preparing the lentils and pasta in advance or using leftovers from another meal since you only need a cup of each.

FOR THE DRESSING

⅓ cup avocado oil

2 tablespoons apple cider vinegar

2 tablespoons water

½ teaspoon dried oregano

¼ to ½ teaspoon sea salt

¼ teaspoon ground black pepper

2 small fresh basil leaves, chopped

FOR ASSEMBLING

1 cup cooked lentils

1 cup cooked green lentil elbow pasta

½ cup unpeeled chopped cucumber

¼ cup thinly sliced onion

5 to 10 small basil leaves, for garnish (optional)

TO PREPARE THE DRESSING

In a small bowl, whisk together the avocado oil, vinegar, water, oregano, salt, pepper, and basil until everything is well combined. Adjust the seasonings to your preference.

TO ASSEMBLE

Add the cooked lentils and pasta to your serving bowl, and gently toss them together so they are evenly distributed. Top with the cucumbers and onions, drizzle with the dressing, and garnish with the basil leaves (if using).

Transfer to 1 large or 2 small plates and enjoy.

TIP Add some variety to this recipe by switching the elbow pasta to either 100-percent red or 100-percent green lentil rotini, penne, or mini fettuccine pasta.

Creamy Artichoke and Basil Red Lentil Penne Pasta

WEEK 3
Serves 2 to 4
Prep: 5 minutes
Cook: 10 minutes

`QUICK & EASY`

This incredibly creamy and flavorful pasta dish is ready in less than 15 minutes, and the star of the show is the red lentil pasta. It has the same shape and texture of traditional pasta, but it's made with 100-percent organic red lentils (one 3-ounce serving of red lentil pasta has 21 grams of protein).

2 cups red lentil pasta

1¼ cups raw cashews

¾ cup almond milk

1 tablespoon freshly squeezed lemon juice

3 garlic cloves

1 tablespoon nutritional yeast

1 tablespoon avocado oil

½ teaspoon sea salt

¼ teaspoon freshly ground black pepper

1 can artichoke hearts, chopped

1 bunch fresh basil, cut into long strips
(about 1 cup)

Cook the pasta according the package directions.

Meanwhile, prepare the sauce. In a high-speed blender, blend together the cashews, almond milk, lemon juice, garlic, nutritional yeast, avocado oil, salt, and pepper until creamy and smooth.

Transfer the drained pasta to a large bowl with the sauce, artichokes, and basil. Toss gently until well mixed, transfer to 2 large or 4 small plates, and enjoy.

TIP Can't find lentil pasta? Don't worry—you can substitute it with spaghetti squash.

Veggie-Stuffed Portobello Mushrooms

WEEK 2
Serves 2
Prep: 10 minutes
Cook: 20 minutes

QUICK & EASY NUT-FREE

This is a colorful and simple meal made with fresh veggies and portobello mushroom caps. Since 60 percent of a portobello mushroom's weight is water, making it a hydrating food, it goes perfectly with the different bell peppers for a light but satisfying lunch or dinner. You can even add or substitute zucchini, squash, or jalapeños to customize them or for variety. Don't be offset by the black "gills" on the underside of the mushroom—they're harmless and can easily be removed before baking them in the oven.

FOR THE MUSHROOMS

2 large portobello mushrooms

Avocado oil, for rubbing

Sea salt

Freshly ground black pepper

FOR THE STUFFING

½ red bell pepper, diced

½ orange bell pepper, diced

½ yellow bell pepper, diced

¼ cup diced red onion

2 garlic cloves, crushed

2 teaspoons avocado oil

½ teaspoon sea salt

½ teaspoon freshly ground black pepper

Preheat the oven to 350°F. Line a baking sheet with parchment paper.

TO PREPARE THE MUSHROOMS

Quickly rinse and dry the mushrooms. Remove the stems, and using the tip of a spoon, scoop out the black gills. Rub the mushrooms all over with avocado oil, and sprinkle with salt and pepper.

Transfer the mushrooms to the prepared baking sheet, and bake for 15 to 20 minutes, or until the mushrooms are as soft as you like.

TO PREPARE THE STUFFING

Meanwhile, in a small bowl, stir together the bell peppers, onion, garlic, avocado oil, salt, and pepper until well combined.

TO ASSEMBLE

Remove the mushrooms from the oven, and discard any accumulated liquid.

Divide the stuffing mixture evenly between the 2 mushrooms and serve immediately.

TIP You can turn this dish into a salad by cutting up the mushrooms after baking and tossing them with the veggies and your favorite salad green.

Zucchini and Kale Pesto Spaghetti Squash

WEEK 2
Serves 2
Prep: 20 minutes
Cook: 50 minutes

Pesto usually includes basil, pine nuts, and some type of cheese, but this recipe uses zucchini, kale, and cashews for a light and flavorful pesto that goes perfectly with spaghetti squash pasta. The nutritional yeast gives it a "cheesy" flavor and is used as a replacement for Parmesan cheese. You can make the pesto in less than 5 minutes while the spaghetti squash is baking, and then it's ready to serve.

FOR THE SQUASH
1 spaghetti squash
2 teaspoons avocado oil
Sea salt
Freshly ground black pepper

FOR THE PESTO
1 zucchini peeled
2 stalks kale, stemmed
½ cup raw cashews
¼ cup chopped onion
2 tablespoons avocado oil
1 tablespoon freshly squeezed lemon juice
1 tablespoon nutritional yeast
2 garlic cloves
½ teaspoon sea salt

Preheat the oven to 350°F. Line a baking sheet with parchment paper.

TO PREPARE THE SQUASH

Halve the spaghetti squash lengthwise, scoop out the seeds, rub the insides and outer rims of both halves with avocado oil, sprinkle with salt and pepper, and place on a baking sheet. Bake for 45 to 50 minutes, or until tender.

TO PREPARE THE PESTO

Meanwhile, in a food processor, process the zucchini, kale, cashews, onion, avocado oil, lemon juice, nutritional yeast, garlic, and salt until well blended. Adjust seasonings, if necessary.

TO ASSEMBLE

Using a fork, scrape out the insides of the squash into long, pasta-like strands. Transfer to a medium bowl.

Add the pesto, and toss gently until well mixed. Transfer to 2 plates or bowls and enjoy.

TIP The Zucchini and Kale Pesto is so versatile. You can use it as the base sauce for the Veggie Pizza on page 120, toss it with red lentil penne pasta, or use it as a spread in a wrap or even as a dip for fresh veggies.

Wild Rice and Broccoli Bowl with Roasted Garlic Sauce

WEEK 3
Serves 1
Prep: 10 minutes
Cook: 20 minutes

Compared to white rice, wild rice is superior in antioxidants, fiber, and plant-based protein. Make sure you get 100 percent wild rice, which is a black, long-grain rice, and not a wild rice blend. The roasted garlic in the sauce adds a depth of flavor that you won't want to miss.

FOR THE ROASTED BROCCOLI AND GARLIC

1 cup bite-size broccoli florets

6 garlic cloves, peeled

1 teaspoon avocado oil

Pinch sea salt

Pinch black pepper

Pinch garlic powder

FOR THE DRESSING

6 roasted garlic cloves (from above)

1 cup raw cashews

1 cup water

½ teaspoon avocado oil

½ teaspoon apple cider vinegar

¼ teaspoon garlic powder

¼ to ½ teaspoon sea salt

Pinch freshly ground black pepper

FOR ASSEMBLING

1 cup cooked wild rice

¼ cup slivered almonds

2 tablespoons diced onion

½ cup chopped collard greens

Preheat the oven to 400°F. Line a baking sheet with parchment paper.

TO PREPARE THE ROASTED BROCCOLI AND GARLIC

In a small bowl, toss the broccoli and garlic with the avocado oil to coat. Season with the salt, pepper, and garlic powder, and transfer to the prepared baking sheet.

Roast the broccoli and garlic for 15 to 20 minutes, or until the broccoli gets soft and slightly crispy.

TO PREPARE THE DRESSING

In a high-speed blender, blend together the roasted garlic cloves, cashews, water, avocado oil, vinegar, garlic powder, salt, and pepper until creamy and smooth. Adjust the seasonings, if necessary.

TO ASSEMBLE

In a serving bowl, stir together the cooked rice with the roasted broccoli, almond slivers, onion, and collard greens. Stir in the dressing and enjoy.

TIP Substitute the collard greens with chopped kale or your favorite alkaline leafy green.

Spicy Cilantro-Lentil "Burgers"

WEEK 2
Makes 4 small "burgers"
Prep: 15 minutes
Cook: 30 minutes

`QUICK & EASY`

These mini burgers are a great use of leftover lentils. They hold together well but are a little delicate, so handle them gently. Top them with a red onion slice, an avocado slice, and a light sprinkling of jalapeño for a bit of heat, or even homemade guacamole.

½ cup dry lentils (equals 1 cup cooked)

½ cup almond flour

½ teaspoon sea salt

½ teaspoon freshly ground black pepper

½ cup diced onion

½ cup chopped cilantro leaves

½ to 1 jalapeño, diced

2 garlic cloves, crushed

1 tablespoon coconut flour

1 tablespoon avocado oil

Prepare the dry lentils according to the package directions. Set aside to cool.

In a medium bowl, stir together the cooled lentils, almond flour, salt, pepper, onion, cilantro, jalapeño, and garlic until well combined.

In a food processor, process half of the lentil mixture until it reaches a paste-like consistency.

Return the processed lentil mixture to the bowl with the other half of the mixture, and stir until well combined. The mixture should be very moist, so mix in the coconut flour to help it hold together.

Take one-quarter of the mixture, squeeze it together in your hand, and flatten it with your palms into a small burger. Repeat to make 3 more patties with the remaining lentil mixture.

In a large skillet over medium-high heat, heat the avocado oil. Add the burgers; cook for 4 to 6 minutes on each side, or until they become golden, flipping them gently; and serve.

TIP The Zucchini and Kale Pesto (page 127) is a delicious topping for these burgers.

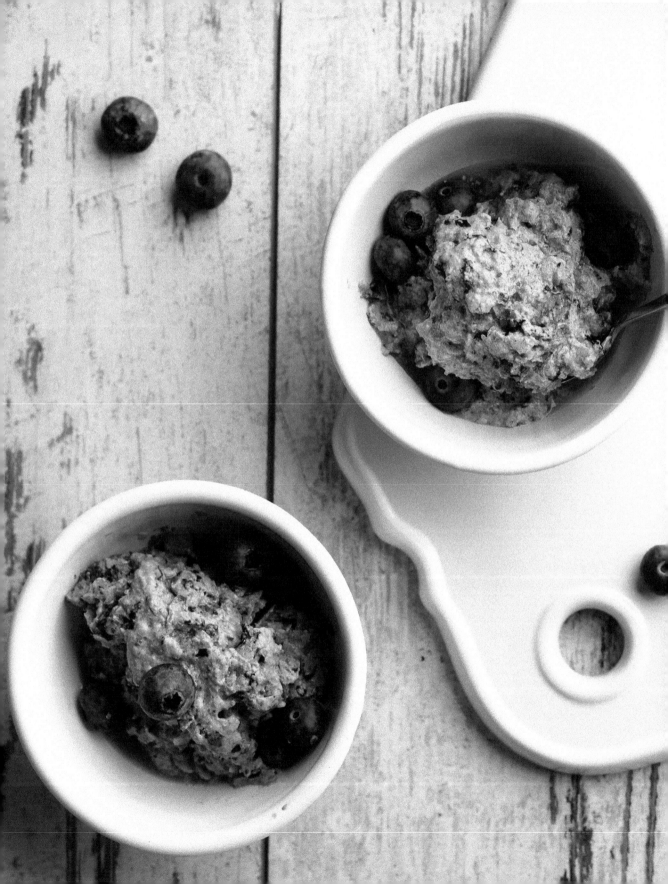

CHAPTER NINE

Delightful Desserts

Flourless Pumpkin Seed Cookies

WEEK 3

Makes 18 to 20 small cookies
Prep: 15 minutes
Cook: 10 minutes

`QUICK & EASY`

These delicate but dense cookies are great with a cup of herbal tea for a healthy afternoon snack. They have a shortbread-like texture and just the right amount of sweetness. You'll want to keep these in the refrigerator because the coconut oil will get soft if they are left out at room temperature.

2 cups raw cashews

½ cup coconut oil

½ cup almond flour

½ cup raw pumpkin seeds

2 tablespoons brown rice syrup

½ teaspoon baking soda

¼ teaspoon sea salt

Preheat the oven to 350°F. Line a baking sheet with parchment paper.

In a food processor, process the raw cashews and coconut oil until the cashews turn into cashew butter. This will take about 10 minutes, and it will go through several different stages (cashews, cashew flour, cashew butter). Stop every 1 to 2 minutes to scrape the sides and make processing easier. This should yield 1 cup of cashew butter.

Transfer the cashew butter to a medium bowl, add the almond flour, pumpkin seeds, brown rice syrup, baking soda, and salt, and stir until well combined.

Scoop a tablespoonful of dough at a time into your hands, and roll into a small ball. Gently press the ball with your palms into a disk. Transfer to the prepared baking sheet. Repeat with the remaining cookie dough.

Bake for 10 to 12 minutes, taking care not to overbake.

Cool completely before removing the cookies from the pan or serving. They will be soft and crumbly right out of the oven but will get firmer after cooling.

Store in an airtight container in the refrigerator to keep the coconut oil from melting.

TIP Make sure you use homemade cashew butter, which has a different consistency than store-bought cashew butter; it will make a difference in this recipe.

Apple Pie Crumble

WEEKS 1 & 4

Makes 6 small pieces
Prep: 10 minutes
Cook: 25 minutes

`QUICK & EASY`

If you love the taste of apple pie, you're in for a treat. This is a really versatile recipe, too, because you can substitute the apple with another alkaline fruit like blueberries, peaches, or even mango; just omit the ground cinnamon powder and lemon juice.

FOR THE APPLE FILLING

1 Braeburn apple, diced small

1 tablespoon brown rice syrup

½ teaspoon ground cinnamon

⅛ teaspoon freshly squeezed lemon juice

FOR THE CRUMBLE

3 tablespoons water

1 tablespoon ground flaxseed

2 cups almond flour

½ cup unrefined whole cane sugar, such as Sucanat

1 tablespoon avocado oil

½ teaspoon ground cinnamon

⅛ teaspoon vanilla bean powder

Pinch sea salt

Preheat the oven to 350°F. Line a 9-by-5-inch loaf pan with parchment paper.

TO PREPARE THE APPLE FILLING

In a small bowl, stir together the apple, brown rice syrup, cinnamon, and lemon juice until well combined. Set aside.

TO PREPARE THE CRUMBLE

In a small bowl, stir together the water and flaxseed to make a flax egg.

In a medium bowl, stir together the flax egg, almond flour, sugar, avocado oil, cinnamon, vanilla bean powder, and salt until well combined.

Take half the crumble mixture, and press it firmly into the bottom of the prepared loaf pan.

Add the apple filling over the crust, spreading it out evenly. Sprinkle the remaining crumble over the apple mixture.

Bake for 20 to 25 minutes and serve.

TIP Want to turn this into an extra-special dessert? Top with a scoop of homemade Whipped Coconut Cream Topping (page 148)!

Chia Seed–Lime Cookies

Makes 12 small cookies
Prep: 15 minutes
Cook: 10 minutes

QUICK & EASY

These tasty little cookies are made without flour, refined sugar, eggs, or butter but are made with only six whole-food ingredients. Homemade cashew butter has a different consistency than store-bought, so there is a little extra step needed to make them. After that, they are ready in less than 15 minutes! As tempted as you might be, make sure you let them cool completely before handling them to give them time to firm up.

2 cups raw cashews

3 to 4 tablespoons coconut oil, divided, as needed

2 tablespoons freshly squeezed lime juice

2 tablespoons chia seeds

2 tablespoons coconut flour

¼ cup brown rice syrup

Pinch sea salt

Preheat the oven to 350°F. Line a baking sheet with parchment paper.

In a food processor, process the cashews and 2 tablespoons of coconut oil until the cashews turn into cashew butter. This will take about 10 minutes, and it will go through several different phases (cashews, cashew flour, cashew butter). Stop every 1 to 2 minutes to scrape the sides and make processing easier. Add 1 tablespoon more of coconut oil at a time, if needed to make creamier cashew butter, but don't exceed 4 tablespoons in total.

Transfer the cashew butter to a medium bowl, and add the lime juice, chia seeds, coconut flour, brown rice syrup, and salt, and stir until well combined.

Scoop a tablespoonful of dough at a time into your hands, and roll into a small ball. Gently press the ball with your palms into a disk. Transfer to the prepared baking sheet. Repeat with the remaining cookie dough.

Bake for about 12 minutes, taking care not to overbake.

Cool completely before removing the cookies from the pan or serving. They will be soft and crumbly right out of the oven but will get firmer after cooling.

TIP Another fun variation of this cookie is to use freshly squeezed lemon juice. Just substitute the lime juice with the same amount of lemon juice.

Cashew Butter Fudge

WEEKS 1, 2 & 3
Makes 16 mini cups
Prep: 5 minutes, plus 2 hours to chill
Cook: None

These mini, bite-size snacks are a perfect midafternoon snack, and the healthy fat from the coconut oil will keep you satisfied. Cashews are an excellent source of magnesium and iron with (1 ounce has 21 percent of your daily value of magnesium and 11 percent of your daily value of iron). Enjoy these plain or with one of your favorite alkaline toppings.

1 cup cashew butter

¼ cup coconut oil (melted/liquid)

2 tablespoons brown rice syrup

Unsweetened shredded coconut flakes, chia seeds, hemp seeds, and/or sesame seeds (optional toppings)

In a medium bowl, stir together the cashew butter, coconut oil, and brown rice syrup until well blended and smooth.

Using a spoon, dividing the mixture evenly among 16 mini muffin cups, filling each cup about three-quarters full.

If desired, top with unsweetened shredded coconut flakes, chia seeds, hemp seeds, or sesame seeds.

Place the muffin cups in the freezer for 1 to 2 hours, or until they are hardened and firm.

Store in the freezer until ready to serve (they will get soft and lose their shape if left out at room temperature).

TIP Add paper muffin cups to a regular muffin cup pan to help keep their shape, and then put the muffin cup pan on a flat baking sheet before putting in the freezer.

Vanilla Bean and Coconut Truffles

WEEK 4

Makes 12 truffles
Prep: 10 minutes, plus 15 minutes to chill
Cook: None

QUICK & EASY

These truffles are simple to make ahead and keep in the refrigerator when you need a quick afternoon snack. They are perfect with a cup of herbal tea, or even as a small after-dinner dessert.

2 cups unsweetened coconut flakes

¼ cup coconut oil

¼ cup brown rice syrup

2 tablespoons coconut flour

2 tablespoons cashew butter

2 teaspoons vanilla bean powder

⅛ teaspoon sea salt

In a food processor, process the coconut flakes, coconut oil, brown rice syrup, coconut flour, cashew butter, vanilla bean powder, and salt until well combined. The mixture should be sticky.

Place the mixture in the refrigerator for about 15 minutes, or until it firms up enough to form a ball shape.

Scoop a tablespoonful of the mixture at a time into your hands, and roll into a small ball.

Store in the refrigerator until ready to serve (they will get soft and lose their shape if left out at room temperature).

TIP Dress up the truffles by rolling them in a small bowl of unsweetened shredded coconut flakes.

Thumbprint Cookies with Blueberry–Chia Seed Jam

WEEK 3

Makes 8 cookies
Prep: 10 minutes, plus 15 minutes to chill
Cook: 10 minutes

These simple cookies are adorned with a colorful fruit topping and are ready in a snap. Blueberries are the perfect pairing with them, and the blueberry Chia Seed Fruit Jam variation (page 146) makes an ideal filling. These aren't overly sweet cookies, so you may want to adjust the sweetener to your preference.

1¼ cups almond flour

3 tablespoons coconut oil, melted

1½ tablespoons brown rice syrup

1 to 2 pinches sea salt

Blueberry Chia Seed Fruit Jam (page 146)

Preheat the oven to 375°F. Line a baking sheet with parchment paper.

In a medium bowl, stir together the almond flour, coconut oil, brown rice syrup, and salt until well combined. The mixture should be very wet. Refrigerate for 10 to 15 minutes, or until firm.

Scoop a tablespoonful of dough at a time and flatten into a disk with your hands. Smooth the outer edges with your fingertips. Press your thumb in the center to make the "thumbprint" indention, and place on the prepared baking sheet. Repeat with the remaining dough.

Bake for about 10 minutes, taking care to not overbake.

Remove the cookies from the oven, and after they cool a bit, repeat the "thumbprint" indention process, if needed. Allow to cool completely before removing from the pan or adding the chia seed fruit topping.

Fill the thumbprint indentions with the blueberry Chia Seed Fruit Jam and serve.

TIP Make several batches of the cookies, and fill each batch with a different chia seed jam flavor for a colorful presentation or party theme!

Blueberry-Banana
Ice Cream

WEEKS 1 & 3

Serves 2

Prep: 5 minutes

Cook: None

`QUICK & EASY` `NUT-FREE`

If you've never tried the popular "nice cream" that's all the rage, you may find it hard to believe that something as simple as a frozen banana can be transformed into a soft serve–type frozen treat. All you need is frozen bananas and your favorite alkaline fruit (such as blackberries, cherries, kiwi, mango, pineapple, strawberries, or peaches) or toppings (such as unsweetened shredded coconut, sliced almonds, and/or hemp seeds).

2 bananas, sliced and frozen

1 cup blueberries

In a food processor, process the frozen bananas pieces and blueberries until the mixture reaches a soft serve–type consistency. Serve immediately.

TIP Always keep at least two sliced bananas in your freezer at all times so you can make this recipe at a moment's notice!

Cinnamon Cashews

WEEKS 2, 3 & 4
Serves 4 to 6
Prep: 5 minutes
Cook: 10 minutes

QUICK & EASY

Typically, sugared cinnamon nuts are made with white, refined sugar and even sometimes egg whites, which is used as a binder to hold the sugar onto the nuts. This healthier version is made with only 4 ingredients and uses water as a binder and unrefined whole cane sugar as the sweetener. These are great to eat as a snack or as a topping on a salad.

½ cup water

½ cup unrefined whole cane sugar, such as Sucanat

¼ teaspoon ground cinnamon

¼ teaspoon vanilla bean powder

1½ cups raw cashews

Line a baking sheet with parchment paper.

In a small saucepan over medium-low heat, stir together the water, sugar, cinnamon, and vanilla bean powder until the sugar is dissolved.

Add the cashews, increase the heat to medium-high, and cook, stirring continuously, for 4 to 6 minutes. Do not leave unattended, as the sugary liquid will begin to thicken and eventually stick to the cashews.

Once all the liquid is gone, remove from the heat and spread evenly onto the prepared baking sheet. Break apart the cashews to dry as individual pieces, or leave some together as clusters.

TIP For a little variety, substitute the cashews with raw almonds.

Chewy Nut and Seed Bars

WEEKS 1, 2 & 3

Makes 8 bars or 16 squares
Prep: 5 minutes
Cook: 25 minutes, plus 45 minutes to cool
Total: 1 hour, 15 minutes

These chewy snack bars may remind you of a popular store-bought nut and seed bar, but this homemade version is so much better. They're made with a variety of alkaline nuts and seeds and are held together with the unrefined whole cane sugar sweetener and brown rice syrup. You can cut them into a traditional bar shape or make smaller portions by cutting them into squares.

¾ cup raw cashews

¾ cup raw almonds

½ cup raw pumpkin seeds

½ cup sesame seeds

½ cup hemp seeds

½ cup unrefined whole cane sugar, such as Sucanat

¼ cup brown rice syrup

1 teaspoon vanilla bean powder

1 teaspoon ground cinnamon

Pinch sea salt

Preheat the oven to 350°F. Line an 8-by-8-inch baking pan with parchment paper.

In a medium bowl, stir together the cashews, almonds, and pumpkin, sesame, and hemp seeds.

In a small saucepan over medium-low heat, stir together the sugar, brown rice syrup, vanilla bean powder, cinnamon, and salt until the sugar dissolves.

Quickly pour the sugar mixture into the bowl with the nuts and seeds and stir until all the nuts and seeds are covered.

Quickly transfer the mixture to the prepared baking pan, flattening it firmly and evenly into the bottom of the pan with your hands.

Bake for 18 to 20 minutes.

Cool completely for 30 to 45 minutes before cutting and serving.

TIP This recipe would also be great for a quick on-the-go breakfast!

Pear Nachos with Sweetened Almond Butter Drizzle

WEEKS 2 & 4
Serves 1
Prep: 5 minutes
Cook: None

QUICK & EASY

This fun dessert requires a firm pear for easy pick-up when dipping. You can drizzle almond butter over the pears or dip them into it. Pears aren't an overly sweet fruit, so just adjust the amount of sweetener in the drizzle to your preference.

1 pear, unpeeled and sliced

2 tablespoons almond butter

2 to 3 teaspoons unrefined whole cane sugar, such as Sucanat

⅛ teaspoon vanilla bean powder

⅛ teaspoon ground cinnamon

1 to 2 tablespoons water, if needed

1 to 2 teaspoons hemp seeds

1 to 2 teaspoons unsweetened shredded coconut flakes

1 tablespoon slivered almonds

Arrange the pear slices on a serving platter.

To prepare the drizzle, in a small bowl, stir together the almond butter, sugar, vanilla bean powder, and cinnamon until well combined. Depending on the thickness of your almond butter, you may need to add 1 to 2 tablespoons of water to thin it out, but only add enough to make it thin enough to drizzle.

Drizzle the almond butter mixture over the sliced pears; garnish with the hemp seeds, coconut flakes, and almonds; and enjoy. Use any extra drizzle to dip the pear slices in.

TIP Swap out the pear with an apple for a sweeter dessert.

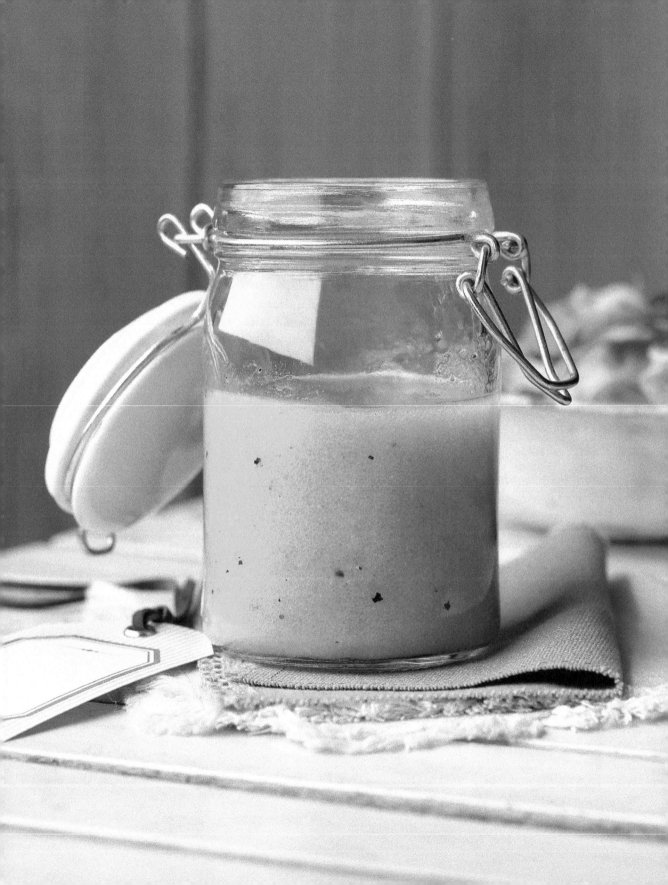

CHAPTER TEN

Kitchen Staples

Nondairy Sour Cream

Makes 2 cups
Prep: 5 minutes, plus 20 minutes to soak
Cook: None

QUICK & EASY

A nondairy sour cream may seem too good to be true, but apple cider vinegar and lemon juice deliver the same tartness as dairy. If you soak the cashews before adding them to your blender, they will blend much more easily and you will get a creamier consistency. You don't have to do it, but it'll make your life a whole lot easier.

1 cup raw cashews

½ cup water, plus more if needed

¼ cup freshly squeezed lemon juice

1 tablespoon apple cider vinegar

½ teaspoon sea salt

In a medium bowl with enough room-temperature water to cover them, soak the cashews for 15 to 20 minutes. Drain and rinse.

In a high-speed blender, blend the soaked cashews, water, lemon juice, vinegar, and salt until creamy and smooth. Add more water if needed, a little at a time, to get the consistency you prefer.

Store in an airtight glass container in the refrigerator.

TIP If the sour cream thickens after refrigeration, add 1 tablespoon of water and stir well to thin it out.

Cashew Cheese Sauce

Makes 1½ cups
Prep: 5 minutes, plus 20 minutes to soak
Cook: None

QUICK & EASY

This sauce is a must-have kitchen staple in any dairy-free kitchen! It works as a dip for veggies, poured over steamed broccoli or cauliflower, drizzled over wraps, or even in a salad. You can even spice it up by adding a little ground chipotle powder. Soaking the cashews before making the sauce is optional, but it will make the sauce extra creamy and smooth and is definitely worth the extra time.

1 cup raw cashews

1 cup almond milk

½ cup nutritional yeast

½ teaspoon sea salt

In a medium bowl with enough room-temperature water to cover them, soak the cashews for 15 to 20 minutes. Drain and rinse.

In a high-speed blender, blend the soaked cashews, almond milk, nutritional yeast, and salt until creamy and smooth.

Store in an airtight glass container in the refrigerator.

TIP If you want to give your cheese sauce a yellow/orange color like traditional cheese, just add 1 to 2 pinches of ground turmeric.

Chia Seed Fruit Jam

Makes 1 cup
Prep: 5 minutes
Cook: None

QUICK & EASY   NUT-FREE

These healthy and simple jams deliver on the taste front with fresh fruit as the main star. The chia seeds add almost the same thickness as a traditional jam. And, you have complete control over the sweetness, depending on the type of fruit you use and the amount of sweetener you add.

1½ cups alkaline fruit (chopped mango, blueberries, chopped strawberries, blackberries, etc.)

¼ cup chia seeds

1 to 2 tablespoons unrefined whole cane sugar, such as Sucanat

In a food processor, process the fruit, chia seeds, and sugar until well blended. Adjust the sweetener, if necessary.

Store extra chia jam in an airtight container in the refrigerator.

TIP Glass mason jars are excellent to use for storing your chia seed jam.

Cashew and Almond Butters

QUICK & EASY

Makes 1 to 1½ cups
Prep: 15 minutes for cashew;
20 minutes for almond
Cook: None

Homemade nut butters are amazing and really easy to make—all you need is patience. It's exciting to watch the nuts go from full nuts to flour, to nut paste, to nut butter. Your reward for patience is fresh, creamy nut butters made with ingredients you decide on.

FOR CASHEW BUTTER

3 cups raw cashews

2 tablespoons coconut oil

FOR ALMOND BUTTER

3 cups raw almonds

3 tablespoons coconut oil

1 to 2 pinches sea salt

FOR CASHEW BUTTER

In a food processor, process the cashews on high until they change to a nut butter, about 15 minutes. Stop and scrape the sides every minute or so to help the processing along.

After about 8 minutes, the nuts should have a paste-like consistency. Add the coconut oil, and continue to process for another 7 to 8 minutes, or until creamy and smooth.

Store in an airtight container.

FOR ALMOND BUTTER

In a food processor, process the almonds on high until they change to a nut butter, about 20 minutes. Stop and scrape the sides every minute or so to help the processing along. After about 10 minutes, the nuts should have a wet, crumbly texture.

Add the coconut oil and salt, and continue to process for another 10 minutes, or until creamy and smooth.

Store in an airtight container.

TIP Glass mason jars are perfect for storing your nut butters.

Whipped Coconut Cream Topping

Makes ¾ cup
Prep: 10 minutes, plus overnight to chill
Cook: None

QUICK & EASY **NUT-FREE**

This simple dairy-free whipped topping can be ready soon after the coconut milk comes out of the refrigerator. You can use this whipped topping on anything that you would normally use a store-bought version for, like Blueberry and Chia Seed Cobbler (page 63) or Apple Pie Crumble (page 133).

1 (13.5-ounce) can full-fat coconut milk

2 tablespoons unrefined whole cane sugar, such as Sucanat

1 to 2 pinches vanilla bean powder

Put the coconut milk in the back of the refrigerator to chill overnight, and up to 24 hours.

Open the can. The top half will be solid (coconut fat) and the bottom half will be liquid. Add the fat solids to a mixing bowl (save the liquid for another use, like a smoothie). Mix on high speed for 2 to 3 minutes, or until peaks form.

Add the sugar and stir it in gently, by hand, until well blended, taking care not to overstir, softening the mixture.

TIP Always keep 1 to 2 cans of coconut milk in the back of your refrigerator so you can make this at a moment's notice.

Basic Vinaigrette Dressing with Variations

Makes ½ to 1 cup
Prep: 5 minutes
Cook: 5 minutes

`QUICK & EASY` `NUT-FREE`

Homemade vinaigrettes are really easy to make and can brighten up any salad with their tangy flavors. Because many common vinegars are acidic, it's helpful to have a variety of flavors to brighten up your dressings. The base of a good vinaigrette is usually one part acid to three parts oil. From there, you can customize it depending on the other ingredients you add, like citrus fruit or fresh herbs. This recipe offers a basic vinaigrette with a few variations to get you started. The method is the same for all three sets of ingredients.

FOR THE BASIC VINAIGRETTE

¾ cup avocado oil

1½ tablespoons apple cider vinegar

1 tablespoon diced shallot

Pinch sea salt

Pinch ground black pepper

FOR THE STRAWBERRY AND LIME VARIATION

¼ cup strawberries

¼ cup avocado oil

¼ cup freshly squeezed lime juice

1 tablespoon brown rice syrup

Pinch sea salt

Pinch ground black pepper

FOR THE LEMON AND THYME VARIATION

¾ cup avocado oil

1½ tablespoons apple cider vinegar

Juice and zest of 1 large lemon

1 tablespoon diced shallot

1 tablespoon chopped fresh thyme leaves

Pinch sea salt

Pinch ground black pepper

In a small bowl, whisk together all ingredients for the vinaigrette dressing of your choice until well combined. Adjust seasonings to your preference.

Store in an airtight container in the refrigerator.

TIP To get the maximum flavor from the ingredients, make sure you use fresh herbs, seasonings, and fruit.

Roasted Garlic

Makes 1 head
Prep: 5 minutes
Cook: 45 minutes

NUT-FREE

Roasted garlic should be a key staple ingredient in every cook's kitchen because the difference it makes in a dish is amazing. It has a strong aromatic flavor that can totally transform a recipe. Instead of aluminum foil, this method shows you how to roast garlic without it. Unbleached paper muffin cups hold the garlic heads perfectly and keep the avocado oil from spilling out.

1 garlic head
1 teaspoon avocado oil
Pinch sea salt

Preheat the oven to 375°F.

Remove the outer papery layer of the garlic head. Cut the top off (the end with the tip), and place the entire garlic head in a paper muffin cup in a muffin pan. Drizzle with the avocado oil, making sure it's evenly distributed in all the crevices, and sprinkle with the salt.

Roast for 45 minutes. Cool until easy to handle.

Gently squeeze or peel each clove out of the paper shell. Use in any recipe that calls for roasted garlic.

TIP Save time by roasting several heads of garlic at once and freezing. To freeze, remove the roasted cloves from their skins, spread evenly on a baking pan, and place in the freezer. After they are frozen, transfer to a freezer-safe container.

Nondairy Tzatziki Sauce

Makes 2 cups
Prep: 5 minutes
Cook: None

QUICK & EASY

Tzatziki sauce is a versatile, light, and creamy sauce. In this recipe, cashews and lemon juice replace the traditional yogurt base to get those classic silky and tart flavors. The sauce is perfection as a salad dressing, over roasted veggies, or as a dip for fresh veggies.

1 cup raw cashews

½ cup water

1 cucumber, peeled and sliced

2 garlic cloves

4 tablespoons freshly squeezed lemon juice

2 tablespoons tahini

3 tablespoons chopped fresh dill, divided

1 tablespoon chopped fresh parsley leaves

½ to ¾ teaspoon sea salt

⅛ teaspoon freshly ground black pepper

In a high-speed blender, blend together the cashews, water, cucumber, garlic, lemon juice, tahini, 1 tablespoon of dill, and the parsley, salt, and pepper until creamy and smooth. Adjust the seasonings, if necessary.

Transfer to a small bowl, and stir in the remaining 2 tablespoons of the dill.

Store in an airtight container in the refrigerator.

TIP Fresh dill will give you optimum flavor, but you could also substitute dried dill.

Chimichurri Sauce

Makes ½ cup
Prep: 5 minutes
Cook: None

QUICK & EASY **NUT-FREE**

Chimichurri is a popular sauce that's traditionally used with grilled meat, but the strong garlic and herb flavor makes it a perfect plant-based condiment. It can be used as a salad dressing, wrap spread, pasta sauce, over roasted veggies, drizzled over a baked potato, or even to dip fresh veggies in. It's a perfect sauce to keep on hand at all times.

2 handfuls fresh parsley leaves

1 handful fresh cilantro leaves

3 garlic cloves

¼ cup avocado oil

2 tablespoons apple cider vinegar

1 teaspoon red pepper flakes

¼ teaspoon sea salt

½ teaspoon freshly ground black pepper

In a blender, blend together the parsley, cilantro, garlic, avocado oil, vinegar, red pepper flakes, salt, and pepper until well combined. Adjust seasonings, if necessary.

Store in an airtight container in the refrigerator.

TIP If you're not making it to use right away, the sauce will marinate in the refrigerator for up to 2 days.

Almond and Coconut Milks

Makes ½ cup
Prep: 5 minutes
Cook: None

QUICK & EASY

Store-bought plant-based milks are very convenient, but they can sometimes be expensive and have added ingredients. These simple recipes will show you how to make homemade almond milk and coconut milk using just two ingredients. You can use these milks in any recipe that you'd use regular milk for, like smoothies, sauces, soups, dressings, and desserts.

FOR THE ALMOND MILK

4 cups water

1 cup raw almonds

FOR THE COCONUT MILK

3 cups hot (not boiling) water

2 cups unsweetened large coconut flakes

FOR THE ALMOND MILK

In a high-speed blender, blend the water and almonds for 2 to 3 minutes.

Strain the almond mixture through a nut-milk bag into a medium bowl. Using your hands, squeeze or wring out any remaining milk.

Store the milk in an airtight container in the refrigerator.

FOR THE COCONUT MILK

In a blender, blend the hot water and coconut flakes for 2 to 3 minutes.

Strain the coconut mixture through a nut-milk bag and into a medium bowl. Using your hands, squeeze or wring out any remaining milk (depending on how hot the water is, you may have to let it cool before touching the nut-milk bag).

Store the milk in an airtight container in the refrigerator.

TIP The milks will separate some in the refrigerator, but just give them a quick stir before using.

Acid-Alkaline Ratings Charts

Food	High Alkaline	Medium Alkaline	Low Alkaline	Low Acid	Medium Acid	High Acid
ALCOHOLIC BEVERAGES						
Beer					●	
Wine, red					●	
VINEGAR AND OIL						
Apple cider vinegar		●				
Avocado oil			●			
Balsamic vinegar				●		
Coconut oil			●			
Olive oil			●			
BEANS AND LEGUMES						
Adzuki beans				●		
Baked beans, vegetarian				●		
Black beans				●		

Food	High Alkaline	Medium Alkaline	Low Alkaline	Low Acid	Medium Acid	High Acid
BEANS AND LEGUMES *continued*						
Chickpeas				●		
Edamame			●			
Great Northern beans				●		
Kidney beans				●		
Lentils		●				
Lima beans				●		
Navy beans				●		
Peanuts					●	
Peas, fresh green				●		
Peas, split green and yellow				●		
Pinto beans				●		
Snow peas			●			
Soybeans						●
String beans				●		
Tofu						●

Food	High Alkaline	Medium Alkaline	Low Alkaline	Low Acid	Medium Acid	High Acid
BEEF/PORK						
Bacon						●
Frankfurters						●
Hamburgers						●
Steak (steaks, roasts, etc.)						●
BERRIES						
Blackberries	●					
Blueberries		●				
Cherries		●				
Raspberries	●					
Strawberries	●					
BEVERAGES						
Apple juice, unsweetened			●			
Carrot juice				●		
Coconut milk, can or carton		●				

Food	High Alkaline	Medium Alkaline	Low Alkaline	Low Acid	Medium Acid	High Acid
BEVERAGES *continued*						
Coffee, regular					●	
Coffee, espresso						●
Cola						●
Grape juice			●			
Grapefruit juice		●				
Milk, 1% fat				●		
Milk, nonfat				●		
Milk, almond unsweetened			●			
Milk, rice					●	
Milk, soy						●
Orange juice			●			
Tea, black				●		
Tea, green			●			
Tea, herbal			●			

Food	High Alkaline	Medium Alkaline	Low Alkaline	Low Acid	Medium Acid	High Acid
BREAD						
Bagel, plain						●
English muffins						●
Matzo, white flour						●
Pita, whole wheat flour					●	
Pumpernickel					●	
100% rye bread					●	
Tortillas, corn					●	
Tortillas, white flour						●
Whole wheat bread					●	
DAIRY PRODUCTS						
American cheese						●
Cheddar cheese						●
Cottage cheese					●	
Cream cheese					●	

Food	High Alkaline	Medium Alkaline	Low Alkaline	Low Acid	Medium Acid	High Acid

DAIRY PRODUCTS *continued*

Food	High Alkaline	Medium Alkaline	Low Alkaline	Low Acid	Medium Acid	High Acid
Egg, white only				●		
Egg, whole				●		
Mozzarella cheese						●
Swiss cheese						●

FISH

Food	High Alkaline	Medium Alkaline	Low Alkaline	Low Acid	Medium Acid	High Acid
Bass					●	
Catfish					●	
Crab					●	
Flounder					●	
Grouper					●	
Salmon					●	
Shrimp						●
Tuna					●	

Food	High Alkaline	Medium Alkaline	Low Alkaline	Low Acid	Medium Acid	High Acid
FLOURS						
Almond flour			●			
Amaranth flour				●		
Barley flour					●	
Buckwheat flour				●		
Millet flour				●		
Oat flour			●			
Rice flour, brown				●		
Wheat flour, white						●
Wheat flour, whole					●	
GRAINS						
Barley, whole grain					●	
Bulgur wheat					●	
Corn					●	
Cornmeal					●	
Freekeh				●		

Food	High Alkaline	Medium Alkaline	Low Alkaline	Low Acid	Medium Acid	High Acid
GRAINS *continued*						
Kasha (buckwheat groats)				●		
Millet				●		
Oat bran					●	
Polenta					●	
Quinoa			●			
Rice, brown				●		
Rice, white					●	
Rice, wild			●			
Wheat, unrefined				●		
FRUITS						
Apple		●				
Apricot		●				
Avocado		●				
Banana		●				

Food	High Alkaline	Medium Alkaline	Low Alkaline	Low Acid	Medium Acid	High Acid
FRUITS *continued*						
Cantaloupe	●					
Coconuts			●			
Date				●		
Fig				●		
Grapefruit		●				
Grapes		●				
Kiwi fruit	●					
Lemon		●				
Mango	●					
Orange		●				
Papaya	●					
Peach		●				
Pineapple	●					
Plum				●		
Pomegranate					●	

Food	High Alkaline	Medium Alkaline	Low Alkaline	Low Acid	Medium Acid	High Acid
FRUITS *continued*						
Tomato				●		
Watermelon	●					

HERBS AND SPICES

Food	High Alkaline	Medium Alkaline	Low Alkaline	Low Acid	Medium Acid	High Acid
Basil		●				
Cilantro		●				
Cinnamon		●				
Cumin		●				
Curry				●		
Dill		●				
Ginger root	●					
Oregano		●				
Paprika	●					
Pepper - black		●				
Salt						●

Food	High Alkaline	Medium Alkaline	Low Alkaline	Low Acid	Medium Acid	High Acid
NUT BUTTERS						
Almond butter			●			
Cashew butter		●				
Peanut butter					●	
NUTS AND SEEDS						
Almonds			●			
Cashews		●				
Chia seeds			●			
Flaxseed			●			
Hazelnuts						●
Hemp seeds			●			
Macadamia nuts			●			
Peanuts					●	
Pecans					●	
Pistachio nuts					●	

Food	High Alkaline	Medium Alkaline	Low Alkaline	Low Acid	Medium Acid	High Acid
NUTS AND SEEDS *continued*						
Pumpkin seeds	●					
Sunflower seeds			●			
Walnuts						●

PASTA

Food	High Alkaline	Medium Alkaline	Low Alkaline	Low Acid	Medium Acid	High Acid
Spaghetti, rye					●	
Spaghetti, white flour						●
Spaghetti, whole wheat flour					●	

POULTRY

Food	High Alkaline	Medium Alkaline	Low Alkaline	Low Acid	Medium Acid	High Acid
Chicken					●	
Duck					●	
Turkey					●	

Food	High Alkaline	Medium Alkaline	Low Alkaline	Low Acid	Medium Acid	High Acid
ROOT VEGETABLES						
Cassava		●				
Taro		●				
Yucca		●				
Beets		●				
SWEETENERS						
Agave nectar		●				
Artificial, aspartame					●	
Artificial, saccharin					●	
Corn syrup						●
Honey				●		
Maple syrup				●		
Molasses		●				
Stevia				●		
Sugar, brown						●
Sugar, white						●

Food	High Alkaline	Medium Alkaline	Low Alkaline	Low Acid	Medium Acid	High Acid
Artichokes		●				
Asparagus	●					
Bell peppers		●				
Broccoli		●				
Brussels Sprouts			●			
Cabbage		●				
Carrots, conventional				●		
Carrots, organic			●			
Cauliflower		●				
Celery		●				
Chard, Swiss				●		
Corn					●	
Cucumbers			●			
Eggplant		●				
Kale	●					

VEGETABLES

Food	High Alkaline	Medium Alkaline	Low Alkaline	Low Acid	Medium Acid	High Acid
VEGETABLES *continued*						
Leeks		●				
Lettuce, arugula		●				
Lettuce, iceberg		●				
Lettuce, red leaf		●				
Lettuce, rocket		●				
Lettuce, romaine		●				
Mushrooms			●			
Mustard greens	●					
Okra		●				
Onions	●					
Parsnips	●					
Potato, white		●				
Potato, sweet	●					
Radishes	●					
Scallions		●				

Food	High Alkaline	Medium Alkaline	Low Alkaline	Low Acid	Medium Acid	High Acid

VEGETABLES *continued*

Food	High Alkaline	Medium Alkaline	Low Alkaline	Low Acid	Medium Acid	High Acid
Spinach				●		
Squash, winter		●				
Squash, summer		●				
Zucchini		●				
Yams	●					

WATER

Food	High Alkaline	Medium Alkaline	Low Alkaline	Low Acid	Medium Acid	High Acid
Bottled mineral, Evian			●			
Bottled mineral, Fiji			●			
Tap, chlorinated					●	

MISCELLANEOUS

Food	High Alkaline	Medium Alkaline	Low Alkaline	Low Acid	Medium Acid	High Acid
Baking chocolate						●
Barbeque sauce					●	
Brownies						●
Butter				●		

Food	High Alkaline	Medium Alkaline	Low Alkaline	Low Acid	Medium Acid	High Acid
MISCELLANEOUS *continued*						
Burrito, with beef						●
Burrito, with chicken						●
Cheesecake						●
Potato chips						●
Croutons						●
Donuts						●
Horseradish	●					
Hummus				●		
Ketchup					●	
Mayonnaise				●		
Mustard					●	
Miso	●					
Popcorn					●	
Pizza						●
Tortilla chips						●

Measurement Conversions

Volume Equivalents (Liquid)

US STANDARD	US STANDARD (OUNCES)	METRIC (APPROXIMATE)
2 tablespoons	1 fl. oz.	30 mL
¼ cup	2 fl. oz.	60 mL
½ cup	4 fl. oz.	120 mL
1 cup	8 fl. oz.	240 mL
1½ cups	12 fl. oz.	355 mL
2 cups or 1 pint	16 fl. oz.	475 mL
4 cups or 1 quart	32 fl. oz.	1 L
1 gallon	128 fl. oz.	4 L

Oven Temperatures

FAHRENHEIT	CELSIUS (APPROXIMATE)
250°F	120°C
300°F	150°C
325°F	165°C
350°F	180°C
375°F	190°C
400°F	200°C
425°F	220°C
450°F	230°C

Volume Equivalents (Dry)

US STANDARD	METRIC (APPROXIMATE)
⅛ teaspoon	0.5 mL
¼ teaspoon	1 mL
½ teaspoon	2 mL
¾ teaspoon	4 mL
1 teaspoon	5 mL
1 tablespoon	15 mL
¼ cup	59 mL
⅓ cup	79 mL
½ cup	118 mL
⅔ cup	156 mL
¾ cup	177 mL
1 cup	235 mL
2 cups or 1 pint	475 mL
3 cups	700 mL
4 cups or 1 quart	1 L

Weight Equivalents

US STANDARD	METRIC (APPROXIMATE)
½ ounce	15 g
1 ounce	30 g
2 ounces	60 g
4 ounces	115 g
8 ounces	225 g
12 ounces	340 g
16 ounces or 1 pound	455 g

The Dirty Dozen and The Clean Fifteen

A nonprofit environmental watchdog organization called Environmental Working Group (EWG) looks at data supplied by the US Department of Agriculture (USDA) and the Food and Drug Administration (FDA) about pesticide residues. Each year it compiles a list of the best and worst pesticide loads found in commercial crops. You can use these lists to decide which fruits and vegetables to buy organic to minimize your exposure to pesticides and which produce is considered safe enough to buy conventionally. This does not mean they are pesticide-free, though, so wash these fruits and vegetables thoroughly.

These lists change every year, so make sure you look up the most recent one before you fill your shopping cart. You'll find the most recent lists, as well as a guide to pesticides in produce, at EWG.org/FoodNews.

Dirty Dozen

Apples	Nectarines	*In addition to the Dirty Dozen, the EWG added two types of produce contaminated with highly toxic organo-phosphate insecticides:*
Celery	Peaches	
Cherries	Spinach	
Cherry tomatoes	Strawberries	
Cucumbers	Sweet bell peppers	Kale/Collard greens
Grapes	Tomatoes	Hot peppers

Clean Fifteen

Asparagus	Eggplant	Onions
Avocados	Grapefruit	Papayas
Cabbage	Honeydew Melon	Pineapples
Cantaloupe	Kiwis	Sweet corn
Cauliflower	Mangos	Sweet peas (frozen)

Glossary

acid/alkaline theory of disease The acid/alkaline hypothesis says that some foods containing acid-forming substances, such as protein from milk, meat, and some plant foods, cause the blood pH to drop or become less alkaline. This effect is then buffered by minerals released from the bone.

acid-ash Acid-ash in food is a residue of the inorganic minerals that form acids in the body. These particles have the capacity of adding hydrogen ions to a liquid solution. An excess of hydrogen ions in a solution makes the solution acid. The more acid in the urine, the more acid-ash in the diet.

acid load Acid load is the excess hydrogen ion production (acid forming residual) after the food has been metabolized by the body.

acidity Acidity describes the level of acid in a substance. It can be characterized as a concentration of free hydrogen ions in it. The lower the pH, the higher the acidity.

alkalinity Alkalinity is the capacity of a substance to neutralize acid solution. The higher the pH, the more alkaline the solution.

antioxidant A substance such as vitamin C or E that removes potentially damaging, oxidizing agents in the body.

ash Foods contain "ash" that, depending on its mineral contents, may be acid-forming or base-forming, having an impact on the acid-base balance in the body.

buffering system of blood pH Buffer systems in the body function to maintain the blood at a steady and optimal pH of 7.40. Our system maintains this balance using three regulatory mechanisms: biochemical, respiratory, and kidney regulation.

buffers A buffer is a solution that prevents a change of pH (change of acidity level) by either adding acidic or basic components.

pH scale The pH scale is a measure of liquid acidity/alkalinity. It ranges from 0 to 14, where 0 is most acidic and 14 is most alkaline. The more acidic, the more hydrogen ions it contains.

phytochemical Any of various bioactive chemical compounds found in plants as antioxidants considered to be beneficial to human health.

PRAL score A calculation of the potential renal acid load of a food. Developed by Thomas Remer and other researchers to assess the acidity of foods and diets. PRAL takes into account the composition of the food, the bioavailability of the different micronutrients and macronutrients (especially protein) of the food, the sulfur content of the food, and the obligatory diet-independent organic acid losses to provide an index of the acid or base load based on a 100 gram portion of the food.

processed foods Processed foods are those that have undergone some processing such as cooking, pureeing, shredding, or blending. Examples are breakfast cereals, processed meats, and cooked and shredded fruits and vegetables.

refined foods Refined foods are those that have had some nutrients purposely removed to obtain a different product. They are different from processed foods where some nutrients may be lost due to heating or freezing. Examples include fiber removed from grains, such as with white rice or white flour.

satiety A feeling of being full after a meal. Foods with a high level of satiety contain protein and fiber.

whole foods Foods that don't purposely have any nutrients removed, although some can be lost through processing such as cooking, drying, blending, or shredding.

whole grain Whole grains are grains that are intact. They are considered as kernels of the grain, which may be cracked, flaked, or ground, but retain the same relative proportions of the starchy endosperm, germ, and bran as the intact grain. Once the bran is removed, the grain is no longer whole.

References

Adeva, M. M. and G. Souto. "Diet-Induced Metabolic Acidosis." *Clinical Nutrition* (2011). 30(4): 416–21.

American Cancer Society. "ACS Guidelines on Nutrition and Physical Activity for Cancer Prevention." (2016). http://www.cancer.org/healthy/eathealthygetactive/acsguidelinesonnutritionphysicalactivity-forcancerprevention. Accessed July 6, 2016.

Andrews, R. "Alkaline Water." *Precision Nutrition*. http://www.precisionnutrition.com/alkaline-water-legit-or-hoax Accessed July 8, 2016.

Centers for Disease Control and Prevention. National Center for Health Statistics. "Hypertension." Updated April 27, 2016. http://www.cdc.gov/nchs/fastats/hypertension.htm Accessed July 5, 2016.

Dawson-Hughes, B., S. S. Harris, L. Ceglia. "Alkaline Diets Favor Lean Tissue Mass in Older Adults. *American Journal of Clinical Nutrition*" (2008). 87(3):662–665.

Fagherazzi, G., A. Villier, F. Bonnet, et al. "Dietary Acid Load and Risk of Type 2 Diabetes: the E3N-EPIC Cohort Study." *Diabetologia* (2013).

Groos, E., L. Walker, J. R. Master. "Intravesical Chemotherapy: Studies on the Relationship Between pH and Cytotoxicity." *Cancer* (1986). 58(6):1199–1203.

National Kidney Foundation. "6 Easy Ways to Prevent Kidney Stones." Updated March 14, 2016. https://www.kidney.org/atoz/content/kidneystones_prevent. Accessed July 5, 2016.

Office of Disease Prevention and Health Promotion. "2008 Physical Activity Guidelines for Americans." http://health.gov/paguidelines/guidelines/summary.aspx Accessed July 8, 2016.

Pizzorno, J., L. A. Frassetto, J. Katzinger. "Diet-Induced Acidosis: Is It Real and Clinically Relevant?" *British Journal of Nutrition* (2009). Doi:10.1017/SO007114509993047.

Remer, T. "Influence of Nutrition on Acid-Base Balance: Metabolic Aspects." *European Journal of Nutrition* (2001). Oct;40(5):214–20.

Remer, T. and F. Manz. "Influence of Diet on Acid-Base Balance." *Seminars in Dialysis* (2000). 13(4):221–6.

Steele, E. M., L. G. Baraldi, M. L. Louzada, J. C. Moubarac, Mozaffarian, et al. "Ultra-Processed Foods and Added Sugars in the US Diet: Evidence from a Nationally Representative Cross-Sectional Study." *BMJ Open* (2016). Doi: 10.1136/bmjopen-2015-009892.

Trinchieri, A., R. Lizzano, F. Marchesotti, G. Zanetti. "Effect of Potential Renal Acid Load of Foods on Urinary Citrate Excretion in Calcium Renal Stone Formers." *Urological Research* (2006); 34(1):1–7.

Vorman, J., M. Worlitschek, T. Goedecke, and B. Silver. "Supplementation with Alkaline Minerals Reduces Symptoms in Patients with Chronic Low Back Pain." *Journal of Trace Elements in Medicine and Biology* (2001);15(2–3):179–183.

Zeratsky, K. "Is Alkaline Water Better for You than Plain Water?" Mayo Clinic. 2016. http://www.mayoclinic.org/healthy-living/nutrition-and-healthy-eating/expert-answers/alkaline-water/faq-20058029 Accessed July 8, 2016.

Resources

Brown, S.E. and L. Trivieri. *The Acid-Alkaline Food Guide – Second Edition: A Quick Reference to Foods & Their Effects on pH Levels.* Mass Market Paperback, 2013.

Health-Diet.us. "Alkaline Diet: PRAL Food Search Database." http://health-diet.us /alkaline-diet/

Remer T, Dimitriou T, Manz F. "Dietary Potential Renal Acid Load and Renal Net Acid Excretion in Healthy, Free-Living Children and Adolescents." *American Journal of Clinical Nutrition* (2003); Vol. 77(5):1255–1260.

Schwalfenberg, G.K. "The Alkaline Diet: Is There Evidence That an Alkaline pH Diet Benefits Health?" *Journal of Environmental and Public Health* (2012); Vol. 2012. Article ID 727630.

Taylor, K. "Basic Acid Alkaline Food Chart Introduction." Foodary Facts.com http://foodary.com/9/basic-acid-alkaline -food-chart-introduction/

Index

CPSIA information can be obtained
at www.ICGtesting.com
Printed in the USA
BVHW050442050619
550138BV00006B/6